# Gut Reloaded

A doctor's guide to transform your gut
microbiome, your health and your life.
Real life stories of faecal transplant at work.

## Dr Paul Froomes

A DOCTOR'S GUIDE TO TRANSFORM YOUR GUT MICROBIOME, YOUR HEALTH
AND YOUR LIFE. REAL LIFE STORIES OF FAECAL TRANSPLANT AT WORK.
Copyright © DR PAUL FROOMES 2018

First published by Zeus Publications 2018
http://www.zeus-publications.com
P.O. Box 2554
Burleigh M.D.C.
QLD, 4220
Australia.

A catalogue record for this
book is available from the
National Library of Australia

All Rights Reserved

No part of this book may be reproduced in any form, by photocopying or by any electronic or mechanical means, including information storage or retrieval systems, without permission in writing from both the copyright owner and the publisher of this book.

This book is a work of non-fiction.

The author asserts his moral rights.

ISBN: 978-1-921919-92-3

# Dedication

This book is dedicated to my wife Caroline

and my children Charlie, Emma and Oscar

who fill me with endless inspiration and joy.

# Gut Reloaded

A doctor's guide to transform your gut microbiome,
your health and your life.
Real life stories of faecal transplant at work.

Dr Paul Froomes

drpaulfroomes.com.au

Melbourne Australia

# Contents

*'[The microbiome is] the ecological community of commensal, symbiotic, and pathogenic microorganisms that literally share our body space and have been all but ignored as determinants of health and disease.'*

Dr Joshua Lederberg
Nobel Prize in Physiology or Medicine (1958) [1]

---

[1] Lederberg J, 2001, ''Ome sweet 'omics: a genealogical treasury of words', *The Scientist*, vol. 15, no. 7.

# Introduction

'Welcome to the 21$^{st}$ century!' I said to my newborn son. 'Yours is the era of obesity, irritable bowel, food allergy and autoimmune disease.' Antibiotics and food chemicals have allowed humanity to trade death from infections for slow decay from chronic disease. And aren't we proud of it? Not if I can help it, my son.

It's now over 150 years since Charles Darwin published his famous paper *On the Origin of Species*. Darwin proved all species evolve according to 'natural selection', which is not so much 'survival of the fittest' but more 'survival of the quickest to adapt'. Human fossil records have given rise to the well-known chart of hominid evolution, beginning with *Homo habilis* around 2.3 million years ago. Until 10,000 years ago, human evolution was fairly static because there were no farms, no crops and no domesticated animals. There were no antibiotics, no pesticides, no food chemicals or colourings, and the nutrient quality of soil, and therefore plants and animals, was richer than it is today. For more than 2.5 million years, human gut bacteria were rich and biodiverse. Our gut contained multitudes of vital probiotic bacteria that had evolved to protect, feed and nurture us.

Somewhere around 10,000 years ago, we humans started to lose our way. During the Neolithic Revolution, *Homo sapiens* hung up their spears and arrows and transitioned from living in nomadic hunter-gatherer bands to agricultural settlements. Our diet changed from foods that were rich in omega-3 fatty acids, such as wild fish, lean meat, berries, seeds and wild vegetables, to crops, grains, fruits, wheat flour, cow's milk, meat from domesticated grain-fed cows, sheep and goats, and sugar from beets and cane. The health of our gut bacteria changed forever.

After 7000 years of human settlement, three disastrous events have occurred. Firstly, modern crops and meats are now 10 to 20 times less nutritional because of over-farming and depleted soil quality. Secondly, food processing has added antibiotics and stripped all the nutritional content out of raw food. Thirdly, our diet relies more and more heavily on sugars like fructose and sucrose, and deep-fried saturated fats.

As a result, stool microbial analysis has shown the population of healthy bacteria living in the human gut has become less and less biodiverse, and bad bacteria have usurped good bacteria. We know this because we finally decided to look closely at our poo and the multitude of bacteria that live in it.

Obesity, irritable bowel syndrome (IBS), food allergies and autoimmune diseases require three things: a genetic predisposition, an environmental trigger and an interface where the environment and a person's genetics meet. What is now clear is that the environmental triggers for irritable bowel syndrome, autoimmune diseases, food sensitivities and obesity are changes in the composition of the bacteria that live in the gastrointestinal tract. The critical interface where bad gut bacteria and our genes meet – where allergy and autoimmune disease begin – is an abnormally permeable intestinal wall. This is known as 'leaky gut'.

As my research into the effect of gut bacteria on disease progressed, it became abundantly clear that the single most important intervention I could give my patients was a program that effectively restored the health and biodiversity of their gut bacteria and improved the function of their gut immune system, gut nervous system and gut barrier. This book is the culmination of the dietary and supplemental approach I have developed through research and my practice as a clinical gastroenterologist, working with faecal transplant and patients with obesity, autoimmune diseases, irritable bowel syndrome, Crohn's disease and ulcerative colitis.

This book will explain three things. Firstly, it will unlock the secrets of how important your gut and the gut bacteria that live in it really are. Secondly, it will explain how your gut bacteria become unbalanced and what relationship this has to illness. We will explore what goes wrong when the gut doesn't function in a normal healthy way. Thirdly, it will show you how you can repair your gut, starting right now. This involves cleansing and reloading your gut with healthy bugs. This book will transform your health in ways you could never have imagined.

Where healthy gut diet books come up short is that they don't outline the critical initial step of cleansing out the bad bacteria that have taken over the gut before reloading the gut with healthy ones. The human bowel is a battleground where a constant power struggle exists between good bacteria and bad. By following the steps in this book, you have the potential to transform your health in ways you could never have imagined.

# Section 1

# The secrets of the gut

# Chapter 1

## Shit, this is serious

Modern medicine is at a crossroads. Debate is raging, and while medical experts argue, patients suffer and die. The greatest paradigm shift of our time in medical thinking is upon us. It's not a new class of drugs, it's not genetic engineering and it's not medical nanobots. The health phenomenon that is sweeping the world can be summed up with just one word: shit. Or, more specifically, the bacteria that live in it.

The current explosion of scientific research on the critical role that gut bacteria (collectively known as microbiota) and intestinal permeability play in human health has the potential to turn our traditional beliefs about health and disease on its head. Yet the pioneers of this research are struggling to have conventional medicine accept their findings.

Every day I hear from patients that their doctor has told them that faecal transplants, probiotics and gut microbiota are all 'bulldust!' This attitude is rife amongst healthcare practitioners, despite the mind-boggling number of medical research studies published in peer-reviewed medical journals that clearly indicate the prominent role that gut microbiota plays in our overall health.

Even as we ignore the potential protective power of the bugs in our bowels, modern medicine is struggling to come up with more potent antibiotics to treat devastating multi-resistant infections. The first was methicillin-resistant *Staphylococcus aureus* (MRSA) and there are now more than 12. Doctors are fighting to invent immunosuppressant drugs to manage the horrible burden of chronic autoimmune diseases like rheumatoid arthritis, type 1 diabetes, multiple sclerosis, systemic lupus erythematosus (SRE), Crohn's disease, psoriasis and primary biliary cirrhosis (PBC). There are over 80 such diseases. All because of ignorance about the importance of maintaining a robust and healthy population of probiotic gut bacteria.

But momentum is gaining. While traditional medicine continues to battle disease using old treatment paradigms, a not-so-quiet gut revolution is underway. It's dramatically changing our understanding of the role our gut plays in causing these conditions and how we can harness our own gut immune system, food and gut bacteria to treat them.

The gut, poo and the magical bacteria that live inside it have rocketed to the forefront of modern medicine as the most exciting new player in the field of health and disease since the discovery of penicillin by Sir Alexander Fleming in 1928.

So, yes. This *is* serious. Studies extolling the myriad health benefits of poo are literally blasting out of the world's leading scientific research laboratories and onto the pages of high-impact scientific journals. You can't pick up a medical journal, attend a gastroenterology conference or watch a health documentary these days without being confronted with evidence proclaiming the magic healing powers of poo.

# Chapter 2

## It's been a long time coming

Nobody likes talking about shit, let alone taking a very close look at it. 'Are you really going to talk about poo? That greasy, offensive-smelling brown excrement that is flushed down the toilet?' The answer is emphatically affirmative.

The traditional view on the subject is this: 'Shit, crap, bog, faeces, dung, poo, stools – it's all just waste'. We are taught from preschool onward that poo is nothing more than the biological digestive equivalent of rubbish. That's why it's called 'taking a dump'.

But let's get technical for a moment. According to *Black's Medical Dictionary*, faeces is 'the remainder of the food after it has passed through the alimentary canal and been subjected to the action of the digestive juices, and after the nutritious parts have been absorbed by the intestinal mucous membrane'. Defaecation or excretion is defined by the Merriam-Webster Medical Dictionary as the process of passing solid waste from the body. The operative word here is 'waste'.

It's no surprise that medicine has ignored poo as a potential treatment. It's smelly, it's ugly, it's 'waste' and we are taught that it is so dangerous that it cannot be touched. The humble act of wiping the bottom with toilet paper is such a threat to our health that we must immediately wash our hands with soap and water to prevent us becoming sick from our own excreta. Poo is unwanted toxic refuse that is fit for nothing but expulsion from the body. I will never forget my grandfather telling me, 'If you don't shit, you die!' when I was only six years old.

Even the act of breaking wind is abhorred. It is viewed as offensive and impolite to those unfortunate enough to be within smelling distance of the fermented gases released from our bowel. While children find it hysterical, adults literally live in fear of the humble fart. Who knows what toxic horrors we are inhaling from that cloud of expelled anal gas?

I once had a friend who was nicknamed 'Arsenic Arse' because he produced the most toxic farts in the history of the Monash University School of Medicine. Etched into my memory is the morning after a big night of watching the footy. We crawled from the football to the pub to a club and ended up at our local kebab house at two a.m. The following morning, still murky-headed from the boozy night before, we fronted up to our nine a.m. lecture. As we tried to focus on cell physiology, Arsenic Arse announced a dire warning. 'Here comes last night's shawarma and extra garlic sauce!' He lifted one buttock cheek off the plastic seat and ripped out one of his famous thunderclap farts. But it wasn't the noise that caused the problem. Row by row, the pervasive vile stench of his gut microbial gases wafted up the lecture theatre. The smell was so visceral and inhuman that it emptied the entire lecture theatre of 145 medical students in a calamity of gagging and crying. The outraged lecturer sent Arsenic Arse to see the university's doctor that day, but his affliction was not cured. They knew nothing of the gut microbiota back in those days. Even now, as a colonoscopist, I have to admit that some bowel gases are so vile and pungent that they can induce a full-blown gag reflex. Thank God for eucalyptus oil.

We haven't always been so terrified of germs and poo. It was only when we decided germs were the root of all disease that we decided to trade body odour for perfumes and antiseptics.

Most of us, depending on our diet and body size, have between six and eleven kilograms of partially digested faecal material loaded with bacteria vigorously fermenting and putrefying in our gut. That knowledge can make even the bravest of us feel uneasy about the colon and everything that comes out of it. The mistake is in thinking that shit is all toxic, festering, poisonous and bad.

The truth is the complete opposite. Your gut, your poo and the bacteria that live in them are part of an important health ecosystem. Your gut is where a number of nutrients and life-sustaining chemicals that keep you alive are made. The once-vilified turd is poised to become the saviour of humanity.

# Chapter 3

## Why are we obsessed with our bowels?

How often have doctors dismissed their patients' ceaseless complaining about the multitude of rumblings, aches, bloats and irregularities of their bowels? If you've ever suffered from what is ignorantly called irritable bowel syndrome (IBS), you know exactly how much misery your bowel can cause.

Studies have shown that around 35% of patients have chronic bowel issues. These bowel groanings are called 'chronic' because no medical drug has been able to fix them. The more you complain about it, the more disinterested your doctor becomes. Finally, you and your gut problems are relegated to that mysterious, unfathomable and untreatable black hole called 'stress-related'. When this happens, you are in no man's land.

Feeling that your bowel troubles are mostly your own fault for being a *stress head,* you probably have enough self-doubt and guilt to stop complaining about it. But unfortunately it doesn't end there. The significant discomfort and impact on your life that ongoing symptoms cause means you will probably turn to any number of allied health practitioners or start trawling the internet.

Why do so many people with gut problems turn to the internet for answers? Because their gut will not stop bothering them. In fact, the gut will keep on complaining more and more and more! It will complain louder and louder until it finally motivates you to go and fix it!

Which brings me to the most important questions. What is up with the gut? Why is it so incredibly persistent and so totally overpowering? And why did I write this book?

I have been asked this many times by my non-medical mates at our monthly male bonding sessions over a beer and a meal at our local Chinese restaurant. (Before you judge me, I can assure you that beer is no threat to your gut bacteria. But I'm the oddball ordering Chinese broccoli and steamed fish, surrounded by the piles of deep-fried dim sum and chicken ribs that my mates tuck into.) Someone always says, 'He's a bum doc. He's obsessed with the arsehole. Don't get him started.' This is followed by riotous cackling and chuckles. Bums and bowels still get a laugh out of 50-year-old men.

But that statement is totally true. I'm a gastroenterologist (a medical bowel specialist), head of the Centre for Irritable Bowel Solutions, head of the Melbourne Faecal Transplant Centre, and the chief medical officer for the Melbourne Gut Microbiome Research Institute. I'm obsessed with bowels. I make my living researching, teaching and treating people with gut problems. I find it fascinating.

And I am not alone. Most of us are obsessed with our bowels. Nature and evolution have ensured it. Each and every one of us has a complex network of nerves, immune cells and chemical messengers that linguistically and metaphorically link our gut to our psyche. We use everyday phrases like 'Go with your gut feeling', 'Stop belly aching', 'She has verbal diarrhoea', 'Let me digest that idea' and 'I can't swallow that notion'. Even my teenage children use bowel expressions when they are texting. 'That's crap', 'She laughed so hard she pooed her pants' and 'You're shitting me.' Hippocrates, the ancient Greek physician who is credited as the father of medicine, said 'all disease begins in the gut'.

When I go out socially and people find out that I'm a gastroenterologist, I invariably get pinned down by somebody who is suffering because of their bowels. Everybody has a unique tale of tummy woe. And apparently, they think, I want to hear every single detail when we are out for dinner.

# Chapter 4

## How important is your gut?

What is the most important organ in your body?

Most people think it's your brain – that one-kilogram noodle in your head that controls everything. But what does your brain really do? Its basic function is to monitor and co-ordinate your body's responses to the information from your sensory organs about the environment you live in. This ensures you adapt to your environment and gives you the best possible chance of survival and reproduction. Your brain is your body's control and command centre, but all it's really doing is responding to what the other organs tell it. For example, when your hand gets too close to a flame, your skin senses the heat but it can't make your hand move. Instead, it sends a message along your nerves to your brain telling it to move your muscles to prevent the skin being damaged. Your brain is just carrying out orders.

What about your skin? Skin is the organ that has the most contact with the environment. It's huge. It has a total surface area of around two square metres, it weighs between five and ten kilograms, it encases you and you feel everything with it. Your skin is basically an interactive pants suit. It acts as a strong and flexible protective outer barrier that reduces water loss and keeps infections out. It is filled with blood vessels, nerve endings, immune cells and melanocytes that protect you from UV damage. The deeper layers store water, fat and nutrients. But it's not your most important organ.

Is it your lungs? You breathe in your environment at a rate of 12 to 20 breaths per minute, which adds up to a staggering 17,000-30,000 breaths every 24 hours. This goes up substantially if you exercise. Your lungs are constantly sampling the environmental gases that you need to sustain yourself (like oxygen) and expelling waste product gas (like carbon dioxide and methane). Despite being packed into the confined space of your chest, your lungs have a total surface area of around 20 square metres – ten times more than your skin. That's a big organ, but it's not the biggest. Your lungs are not your most important organ.

The most important organ of them all is your gut. Your gut, at first glance, is just a long tube that begins at your mouth and ends at your anus. The inside of that tube is basically outside you. You could swallow a stone and it would pass through your entire gut and out your anus without ever entering your blood stream. You never really interacted with the stone at all. Just as a stone tossed at you will bounce off your skin, a swallowed stone will also bounce off your gut. You could literally swallow one end of a piece of string and when it comes out of your anus you could grab each end with your hands and pull it up and down through yourself, flossing your gut.

Your gut is around eight metres long. This tubular organ of digestion is the gateway to your body. It has a surface area of a staggering 40 square metres, all made possible by layers of intricate folding that create tower-like structures called plicae circulare, then villi, then microvilli.

What does this mean? The traditional view is that this structure offers the greatest possible surface area for the absorption of nutrients that keep us alive and functioning. For centuries, this explanation of the gut as simply a mindless absorbent surface has satisfied even the greatest medical minds on the planet. This view, as it turns out, is the greatest over-simplification of them all. It has blinded us to the real purpose of the gut as the master controller of the human being.

Your gut is unlike any other organ. It is equipped with its own special lining, immune system, microbial mass, nervous system and even its own brain.

# Chapter 5

# Gut digestion

I don't deny that one of the primary functions of the digestive tract is to ensure we eat food, break it down and absorb the nutrients that are needed to keep us alive. It does this in several ways. It is the gut that prods us to seek out and enjoy food through a multitude of smell receptors and taste receptors. The gut also drives us crazy with an unpleasant sensation called hunger, which it controls by secreting the potent hunger hormone, grehlin.

The process of digestions starts with the sight or the smell of food. Food-digesting enzymes are actively secreted into your saliva the moment you smell or see your meal approaching. It continues when the food hits your mouth, as digestive enzymes squirt into your mouth and your mouth bacteria begin to break down the food, and digestion ramps up as the food slides down your gullet and drops into your stomach.

The stomach is a hostile environment. It's designed to mechanically grind up partially chewed food and then secrete digestive enzymes to chop up small food particles into microscopic ones. But it also needs acid. The stomach is lined with acid-secreting cells that squirt concentrated hydrochloric acid into the stomach to begin the gastric phase of digestion. Acid is also needed to switch on digestive enzymes. These are produced in a non-active form, so they don't start breaking down the stomach itself, and they can only be activated in the presence of acid.

If the stomach fails to produce sufficient acid, gastric digestion cannot be completed. This is a particular problem when eating meat, which is high in protein and fat. Both fat and protein must be properly broken down in the stomach before moving to the small intestine. If poorly digested meat hits the small intestine, it can't be further broken down into single molecules for absorption. Instead, a slimy, undigested semi-solid lump of meat passes through the small intestine and into the colon, making the person nauseated, bloated, crampy and weak. When the rancid meat slides into the colon the gut bacteria go to work on it, fermenting and putrefying it into a gooey, smelly mess. The resulting flatulence can be stifling and very offensive to the nose.

This is why people who are low acid producers feel ill when they eat meat. Their stomachs don't bring enough acid to the table so they can't digest it properly. This is becoming a major problem nowadays because of the overuse of drugs called proton pump inhibitors (PPI), which are used to treat acid reflux. These drugs are so effective at reducing acid levels in the stomach that they inhibit stomach digestion. To give you a sense of the scale of this potential problem, a recent US study found that PPI drugs were prescribed 269.7 million times from 2006 to 2010.[2] In Australia, we follow the same prescribing patterns as the US. That's a lot of acid suppression.

The next phase of digestion and absorption occurs in the five or so metres of your small intestine. The minute your semi-digested food slurry, or 'chyme', slides from the stomach into the small intestine, the pancreas glands begin squirting out an alkali solution. That's right – as soon as your stomach finishes its acid work, your digestion suddenly switches to alkali digestion. This is because the very thin lining of your small intestine – it's just a single cell thick – can't cope with the amount of acid contained in the food slurry from your stomach without being burnt. The lining has to be thin to allow it to absorb all the nutrients you need to sustain life.

The presence of acid in the chyme that comes out of the stomach induces the rapid release of a hormone called secretin from specialised cells that line the small intestine. Secretin's job is to whip up the pancreas to start pumping out alkaline bicarbonate juice into the intestine to neutralise the stomach acid as quickly as possible. Now the most important phase of digestion can begin.

The fats and protein fragments in the chyme stimulate the release of a messenger hormone called cholecystokinin (CCK) from special neuroendocrine cells of the intestinal lining and the brain. CCK binds to receptors on the stomach, telling it to stop making acid, and the gall bladder, telling it to start contracting and squirting bile into the intestinal soup. It also binds to receptors on the pancreas and tells the pancreas to start secreting pancreatic juice. CCK in the bloodstream also binds to CCK receptors in the part of your brain called the hypothalamus that reduce your appetite. This is designed to make you stop eating, giving your intestine enough time to digest the food and extract all the nutrients before the next wave of semi-digested chyme comes rushing in.

The bile from your gall bladder emulsifies the fats into tiny little droplets that are small enough for the pancreatic juice to break down into basic one-molecule components. Fats are very important: every cell in the body is made of fat. When the fats are small enough, they are absorbed straight into the lymphatic system.

The proteins in the chyme are chopped up by enzymes in the pancreatic juice. Once the proteins have been reduced to single beads, called amino acids, they are gobbled up by amino acids carriers and swept into the gut's bloodstream.

Finally, carbohydrates, which are just long chains of sugars, are pulled apart by a bunch of enzymes called amylases. The single sugar units – glucose, galactose, maltose and the like – are sucked up through diffusion and pumped into the blood stream.

Most people are familiar with lactose, the sugar found in cow's milk. Even though lactose is made up of only two molecules, it is too big to be absorbed by

---

[2]    Gawron AJ et al, 2015, 'Brand name and generic proton pump inhibitor prescriptions in the United States: insights from the National Ambulatory Medical Care Survey (2006–2010)', *Gastroenterology Research and Practice*, vol. 2015, article ID 689531, pp. 1-7.

the digestive tract. An intestinal enzyme called lactase recognises lactose and cuts the bond between the molecules, like a key opening a lock. This frees up the two small sugar molecules – glucose and galactose – which are small enough to be absorbed by the gut.

Many people are born with a gene mutation that switches off the enzyme that breaks down lactose once you hit adolescence. If your body does not make lactase anymore, you are lactose intolerant. Every time you drink cow's milk, the lactose in it passes straight through the small intestine without being properly digested and gets dumped into the colon. Sugars cause havoc in the colon. The bacteria get to work fermenting lactose, which produces lactic acid, water and lots of gas. The sugar itself exerts an osmotic pressure on the colon, causing the outpouring of water. The lactic acid can cause pain and the gas can bloat you like you're carrying a set of triplets. This can bring on abdominal pain, cramping, bloating, distension and diarrhoea.

When the small bowel is finished with your food, it is the turn of your colon (also known as the large bowel). The colon is not as specialised an organ – it's more like a big fermentation vat that houses massive quantities of life-supporting bacteria. Using those bacteria, the colon does some last-minute digestion of fibrous vegetable matter to extract any extra vitamins, antioxidants, electrolytes and minerals that weren't absorbed by the small intestine. Finally, the colon prepares and extrudes waste and non-digested materials.

# Chapter 6

## What's left is just shit, right?

Shit (or faeces, if you prefer the medical term) has offended, revolted, fascinated and amused people since the beginning of human evolution. The medical profession has been brought – kicking and screaming in many cases – to show more than a passing interest in poo by the tireless demands of our patients.

Medicine's major contribution to the understanding of poo problems is the Bristol Stool Chart. (Stool is yet another word for shit.) This chart, which lets doctors appear knowledgeable when discussing faeces, allows us to classify patients' stools as 'too hard', 'too loose' or 'normal' and push them out of our consulting rooms with a laxative, a constipating agent or an assurance that their bowels are fine and they are probably just anxious.

| Bristol stool chart[3] | | |
|---|---|---|
| Type 1 | Separate hard pellet-like lumps | Very constipated |
| Type 2 | Lumpy and sausage-like | Slightly constipated |
| Type 3 | Sausage shaped with surface cracks | Normal |
| Type 4 | Smooth soft sausage-like | Normal |
| Type 5 | Soft blobs with clear cut edges | Lacking fibre |
| Type 6 | Mushy consistency with ragged edges | Inflammation |
| Type 7 | Liquid consistency with no solid pieces | Inflammation |

About 1.5 litres of undigested and partially digested food passes from the small intestine into the colon each day. As the chyme moves through the first half of the colon, large amounts of water and electrolytes are absorbed. Despite this, water continues to make up about 70% of the faecal weight. Water absorption

---

[3]    Heaton KW & Lewis SJ, 1997, 'Stool form scale as a useful guide to intestinal transit time',
    *Scandinavian Journal of Gastroenterology*, vol. 32, no. 9, pp. 920-924.

transforms the fluid chyme into a mushy consistency as it passes through the transverse colon. It solidifies further along its passage down the descending colon.

The average person passes between 100-200 grams of faeces per day – about a cupful. It comes out coated in mucus to ease its passage as it squeezes through the narrow sphincter muscles of the anal canal. Without our sphincter muscles, we'd all be incontinent.

Faecal matter is a complex mix of traces of plant- and animal-based proteins, fats and carbohydrates as well as DNA, gut digestive enzymes, hormones and bile salts. It also has a very high water content – up to 85%. However, gram for gram, the dry weight of your stool is made up of bacteria (30-40%), undigested food and fibre (20-30%), fat (10-20%), inorganic matter (10-20%) and other proteins from food and produced by gut bacteria (2-3%).

Around $10^{14}$ bacteria are excreted in faeces. A decade ago, it was thought that all those bacteria were dead. We now know that the majority of stool bacteria are live. These stool-derived bacteria can be preserved for hours. They can even be frozen and then thawed – and still be alive. It is these precious probiotic bacteria that provide the benefit that comes from faecal transplant.

# Chapter 7

## The gut barrier

One of the reasons the gut is such an important organ is because its massive absorptive surface doubles as a barrier to everything that is not completely digested. Every morsel that you pour down your throat – food, drink, drugs, pesticides, pills, alcohol or poison – goes down the digestive tract pipe and it stays there unless it is digested or absorbed. Anything not used ends up excreted in faeces.

We sample our environment predominantly through our digestive tracts. The 30 tons of food that we eat our way through represents an awful lot of environmental information, some healthy and some dangerous. The information the gut gets from our food and drink determines which of our genes need to be turned on and off to allow us to adapt to our ever-changing environment.

*The intricate job of deciding which molecules are allowed into the body and which aren't is carried out by the single layer of enterocytes that line the gut. Which brings us to the other key function of the gut: to block the absorption of anything but specific nutrients into our bloodstream.*

Enterocytes can do this because every cell is linked to its neighbour by a complex network of proteins known as tight junctions. As recently as 50 years ago, the tight junctions that link these cells were thought of as a kind of extracellular cement forming a rigid, mindless barrier. But, like so many concepts in science, that turned out to be completely wrong. In 1998, scientists discovered that tight junctions contain a complex matrix of proteins and muscle cells that open and close, allowing molecular trafficking to occur between the enterocytes.

Biological studies over the past several decades have shown that tight junctions are dynamic structures, subjected to structural changes that control their function. The movement of molecules between cells is dictated by changes in the permeability of the gut lining. But, as you would expect, the permeability of the gut lining is very well controlled. The spaces between cells are tiny – anything bigger than a single molecule of food will be excluded.

We have a very accurate understanding of tight junctions. They are made up of a network of junctional adhesion molecules (JAM), which are proteins that span the space between the cells. The JAMs are anchored to the cell walls by another set of proteins called the junctional complex. These guys function as a linking scaffolding – one end is attached to the JAMs and the other end is bound to small muscle cells inside the enterocytes. The muscle cells are attached to the bricks and mortar of the enterocytes, and they are able to contract and relax.

One of the most fascinating and significant discoveries related to gut permeability is the discovery of a bacterial toxin called *zonula occludens toxin* (Zot). Zot is secreted by the nasty little pathogen that causes cholera and it opens tight junctions until it is broken down. This simple finding blew open our understanding of tight junctions and gut permeability and led to the discovery that our own enterocytes make a protein very similar to Zot called zonulin.

It turns out that zonulin binds a receptor on the surface of intestinal cells that makes tight junctions open. This is called the zonulin pathway and it is responsible for the movement of fluid, macromolecules and white blood cells into the bloodstream and back again. A healthy functioning gut barrier is essential to prevent the entry of potentially harmful substances into the bloodstream. Anything that cannot be used by the body is recognised as foreign and triggers an instant attack by our immune system. A growing number of diseases are known to involve changes in intestinal permeability, and people affected by autoimmune diseases have high levels of zonulin.[4]

Despite this knowledge, Western medicine is still loath to attach any significance to the part that the gut plays in disease. Understanding the role of the intestinal barrier in the pathogenesis of gastrointestinal disease is the subject of significant research, yet this fails to attract the attention of the medical profession.

---

[4]    Fasano A, 2012, 'Zonulin, regulation of tight junctions, and autoimmune diseases' *Annals of the New York Academy of Sciences*, vol. 1258, no. 1, pp. 25-33.

# Chapter 8

## The gut immune system

Yet another reason the gut is your most important organ is that it has its own dedicated immune system. In fact, 80% of your body's entire immune system is contained in your gut. The gut immune system makes more decisions in one day than the rest of your body does in a whole lifetime. This is hardly surprising when you think about the rubbish dump amount of food we eat our way through in our life. Our intestinal immune system is the first line of defence against the tons of pathogens, bugs and chemicals that we eat all day, every day.

For centuries we believed that the only real function of the intestine is to break down food into its most basic nutrient form. However, with the coming of age of the medical science of immunology, intestinal immune function has hit centre stage. It was discovered that the intestine houses a mass of highly specialised gut immune cells. The main job of this intestinal immune system is to discriminate between beneficial food nutrient, harmless or beneficial bacteria and bad bacteria.

There are two arms to our gut immune system: the innate and the acquired immune systems. They communicate with each other to form a formidable defence force. To prevent our gut immune cells from attacking harmless or beneficial bacteria, both intestinal immune systems have to be trained to ignore probiotic gut bacteria and only go after the bad guys. This is called immune tolerance.

Put simply, the process of deciding whether to fight or to tolerate something in the gut begins with the soldiers of the innate immune system – the first responders of the immune defence team. These cells are literally sitting on the front line of the gut, looking for trouble.

Their first job is to set up a defensive perimeter made up of mucus and an antibody called secretory IgA (sIgA). sIgA seeks out and binds onto the bacteria living in the gut, both good and bad, and anchors them in the outer layer of mucus. This keeps them captive, where they can do the job of digesting tough foodstuffs and manufacturing vitamins and nutrients. It also keeps them away from the delicate enterocyte cells that line our gut.

But we don't want any bacteria – good or bad – sneaking out of the mucus factory and touching our gut-lining cells. Even good bacteria are too irritating if they get too close. As soon as this happens, the gut has to push them back to a safe distance. The gut defensive perimeter is a bit like a fence at the zoo that keeps the lions on one side and the people on the other. If the fence is breached, the people might get eaten and the lions might get shot and killed.

The cells of the gut innate immune system are also constantly sampling the bacteria in the gut mucus factory. They keep a close eye on these bugs because they need to know very quickly if there are potential disease-causing or pathogenic bacteria sneaking into the factory. They gobble up random worker bacteria and present them for inspection to the big boys of the second line of defence: the acquired immune system of the gut. The soldiers of the acquired immune system are called T lymphocytes or, more commonly, T cells. They are the elite commandos of the gut army. They can adapt and equip themselves to fight and kill any enemy. After receiving a signal from the innate cells of the front line, the T cells bring the weapons best suited to fight that specific threat. It's an incredibly responsive and efficient attack force.

The way that the innate cells signal to the T cells is simple. Firstly, they chew up a worker bacteria and then present the specific recognition or identity bits of that bacteria on a presentation board that the T cells are constantly looking at. Secondly, the innate cells gobble up any bits of gut cells that are currently being damaged and put them on the board too. Thirdly, they put out an instruction signal to tell the T cells if they think these bacteria are bad or good.

The T cells read the presentation boards, checking them out for co-stimulatory signals and any signs of damage to the gut. Probiotics are good bacteria that do no damage to our cells, so those presentation boards contain bits of probiotic bacteria, no damage to associated molecules and a signal from the innate immune cells that says 'All good, calm down'. The T cells maintain their relaxed state and move on. They are trained to tolerate these good bacteria.

If the innate cells pick up a bad bug, the presentation board contains the recognition antigens of the bad bug, damage-associated molecules and an instruction signal that says 'Fight'. The T cells go to war. They mobilise their attack force called B cells to make antibodies that recognise, lock on and start attacking the bad bacteria. The threat is terminated.

But when this system goes wrong, autoimmunity occurs.

# Chapter 9

# The gut nervous system

The human gut is so important that it has evolved its own highly sophisticated nervous system. Gut symptoms are common to most people with obesity, allergies, autoimmune diseases and irritable bowel. The gut has only so many ways it can complain to you that something is wrong: pain, cramping, nausea, bloating, abdominal distension, wind, diarrhoea and constipation.

One of the hallmarks of people with unbalanced gut bacteria and leaky gut is oversensitivity of the gut nerves. The gut nerves communicate pain signals to your brain, so oversensitivity ensures discomfort. Doctors call it 'visceral hypersensitivity'.

This has been known since 1973, when it was elegantly demonstrated in human experiments using the infamous anal balloon. Researchers convinced normal people and people with IBS to let them stuff an anal balloon up their bum and blow it up until their eyes watered and they felt pain. The normal subjects didn't complain until the balloon reached 150 ml, but the poor IBS patients reported significant pain when the balloon reached 60 ml. This study proved that patients with IBS were more sensitive to mechanical colonic distension than normal patients. They had a much lower pain threshold and experienced a greater intensity of pain. In practice, this means that even with a low level of bloating and fermentation in the colon, IBS patients feel pain, and it's not in their heads.[5]

Visceral hypersensitivity is mediated by bad gut bacteria. The wrong balance of microbes living in the colon sets off a cascade of neural events. This painful response to colorectal distension was later assessed in rats. The rats were inoculated with faecal microbiota, either from IBS patients who had marked visceral hypersensitivity or non-hypersensitive healthy volunteers. The number of abdominal contractions in response to colorectal distensions was significantly higher in the IBS rats than in the healthy rats.

In mice, it has been shown that a faecal microbial transplant from an IBS-affected mouse to a healthy mouse practically transfers the condition along with it. The formerly healthy mouse exhibits IBS-like hypersensitivity after the transplant.

Visceral hypersensitivity is widely regarded as the reason for the development of symptoms of gastrointestinal disorders, including indigestion and IBS, and abdominal pain is what forces most people to seek help. Pain is the gut's way of alerting you to the fact that things are not right. As long as the gut wall and gut

---

[5] Richie J, 1973, 'Pain from distension of the pelvic colon by inflating a balloon in the irritable colon syndrome', *Gut*, vol. 14, no. 2, pp 125-132.

bacteria are in balance, the gut remains a diligent servant that never bothers you. After all, your gastrointestinal tract is supposed to function at a subconscious level. There is an entire nervous system that operates the machinery of your body at a subconscious level, leaving your brain free to think about more important things. An imbalance in your gut bacteria ramps up the gut nervous system so much that it takes over. Once it's cranked up, it's very difficult to settle.

Let's talk briefly about the nervous system. You have a central nervous system – the brain and the spinal cord – and a peripheral nervous system, which has two parts. The first part, the somatic nervous system, handles all of your voluntary physical sensations and body movements. The somatic nervous system is conscious, meaning that you are always aware of it. It operates through sensory receptors in your skin, which send signals to your brain that activate muscle movements. These simple reflex circuits control your withdrawal reflexes, like when you touch a hot object and quickly jerk your hand away. It's a protective neurological mechanism and you are fully conscious of it.

The second part of the peripheral nervous system, the autonomic nervous system, is connected to your internal organs. It regulates fundamental states of physiology, including your heart rate, digestion, respiration, salivation, perspiration, pupillary dilation, temperature and sexual arousal. These functions are carried out automatically at a subconscious level, meaning your brain is largely oblivious to all work that keeps your bodily functions on track. Most of the work is done through spinal cord arcs that never reach the brain.

This two-part system provides a balance between relaxation and excitation that is needed for us to survive in our environment. It's also necessary for emergency reactions, such as the 'flight or fight' response. The complex network of neural connections that make up your body's nervous system operates at terrific speed. The nerve conduction velocity of the average human nerve has been clocked at around 100 metres per second. That's not too shabby, considering the speed of sound is 340 metres per second. Our reaction times are pretty damn fast.

But, thanks to extensive research, we have now discovered an entirely new nervous system. It has been dubbed the 'second brain' and it is located in our gut.

The enteric nervous system (ENS) is made up of 500 million neurons, which is about the same size as a rabbit's brain. This network of nerves stretches for nine metres and connects everything from your mouth to your anus. Embedded in the wall of the gut, the ENS has long been known to control digestion. It can work both independently of and in conjunction with your brain and, although you are not conscious of your gut 'thinking', the ENS senses environmental threats and influences your response.

'A lot of the information that the gut sends to the brain affects wellbeing, and doesn't even come to consciousness,' says Michael Gershon of the Columbia-Presbyterian Medical Center in New York. 'It is also the original nervous system, emerging in the first vertebrates over 500 million years ago and becoming more complex as vertebrates evolved, possibly even giving rise to the brain itself.'

Digestion is a complicated business, so it makes sense to have a dedicated network of nerves to oversee it. As well as controlling the mechanical mixing of food in the stomach and coordinating muscle contractions to move it through the gut, the ENS also maintains the biochemical environment within different sections of the gut, keeping them at the correct pH and chemical composition needed for digestive enzymes to do their job.

But there is another reason the ENS needs so many neurons. Eating is fraught with danger. The gut has to stop potentially dangerous invaders from getting inside the body. If a pathogen crosses the gut lining, immune cells in the gut wall secrete inflammatory substances like histamine that are detected by neurons in the ENS. The gut brain then either triggers diarrhoea or alerts the brain, which may decide to initiate vomiting. Or both.

You don't need to be a gastroenterologist to be aware of these gut reactions. Think of the subtle feelings in your stomach that accompany emotions such as excitement, fear and stress. For hundreds of years, people have believed that the gut interacts with the brain to influence physical and mental health and disease, yet this connection has only been studied over the last century.

Two pioneers in this field were American physician Byron Robinson, who published *The Abdominal and Pelvic Brain* in 1907, and his contemporary, British physiologist Johannis Langley, who coined the term 'enteric nervous system'. Around that time, it also became clear that the ENS can act autonomously. It was discovered that if the vagus nerve – the main connection with the brain – is severed, the ENS can still coordinate digestion. Despite these discoveries, interest in the gut brain waned until the 1990s, when the field of neurogastroenterology was born.

We now know that the ENS is not just capable of autonomy, but that it also influences the brain. In fact, about 90% of the signals passing along the largest cranial nerve that connects the brain to the body, called the vagus nerve, come from the ENS.[6]

The 'second brain' shares many features with the first. It is made up of various types of neurons and support cells. It has its own version of a blood-brain barrier to keep its physiological environment stable. And it produces a wide range of hormones plus around 40 neurotransmitters, or chemical messengers, that are the same as those found in the brain. In fact, the neurons in your gut are thought to generate as much dopamine as those in your head. Intriguingly, about 95% of the serotonin present in your body at any time is in the ENS.

What are these neurotransmitters doing in the gut? In the brain, dopamine is a signalling molecule associated with pleasure and the reward system. It acts as a signalling molecule in the gut too, transmitting messages between neurons that coordinate the contraction of muscles in the colon. Another neurotransmitter in

---

[6]   Powley TL & Phillips RJ, 2002, 'Morphology and topography of vagal afferents innervating the GI tract', *American Journal of Physiology - Gastrointestinal and Liver Physiology*, vol. 283, no. 6, G1217-G1225.

the ENS is serotonin, best known as the 'feel-good' molecule involved in preventing depression and regulating sleep, appetite and body temperature. But its influence stretches far beyond that. Serotonin produced in the gut gets into the blood, where it is involved in repairing damaged cells in the liver and lungs. It is also important for normal development of the heart, as well as regulating bone density by inhibiting bone formation.[7]

But what about mood? Obviously, the gut brain doesn't have emotions, but can it influence those that arise in your head? The general consensus is that neurotransmitters produced in the gut cannot get into the brain. Nevertheless, nerve signals sent from the gut to the brain do appear to affect mood. Research published in 2006 indicates that stimulation of the vagus nerve can be an effective treatment for chronic depression that has failed to respond to other treatments.[8]

Such gut-to-brain signals may also explain why fatty foods make us feel good. When ingested, fatty acids are detected by cell receptors in the lining of the gut that send nerve signals to the brain. This may not be simply to keep it informed of what you have eaten. Brain scans of volunteers given a dose of fatty acids directly into the gut show they had a lower response to pictures and music designed to make them feel sad than those given saline. They also reported feeling only about half as sad as the other group.[9]

There is also evidence of links between the two brains in our response to stress. The feeling of butterflies in your stomach is the result of blood being diverted away from it to your muscles as part of the 'fight or flight' response. However, stress also leads the gut to increase its production of ghrelin, a hormone that, as well as making you feel hungry, reduces anxiety and depression. Ghrelin stimulates the release of dopamine in the brain. It does this directly, by triggering neurons involved in pleasure and reward pathways, and indirectly, by signals transmitted via the vagus nerve.

Gershon suggests that strong links between our gut and our mental state evolved because a lot of information about our environment comes from our gut. 'Remember the inside of your gut is really the outside of your body,' he says. We see danger with our eyes, hear it with our ears and detect it in our gut. Pankaj Pasricha, director of the Johns Hopkins Center for Neurogastroenterology in Baltimore, points out that without the gut there would be no energy to sustain life. 'The vitality and healthy functioning of the gut is so critical that the brain needs to have a direct and intimate connection with the gut,' he says.

---

[7]   Yadav VK et al, 2008, 'Lrp5 controls bone formation by inhibiting serotonin synthesis in the duodenum', *Cell*, vol. 135, no. 5, pp 825-837.

[8]   Corcoran CD et al, 2006, 'Vagus nerve stimulation in chronic treatment-resistant depression – preliminary findings of an open-label study', *The British Journal of Psychiatry*, vol. 189, p. 282-283.

[9]   Van Oudenhove L et al, 2011, 'Fatty acid-induced gut-brain signaling attenuates neural and behavioural effects of sad emotion in humans', *The Journal of Clinical Investigation*, vol. 121, no. 8, pp. 3094-3099.

# Chapter 10

## Food is dangerous

One of the main reasons the gut is such an important organ is because it has to handle a mind-boggling onslaught of nutrients, chemicals, microbes, toxins and antigens every single day. How much food do you think you munch through in your lifetime? Most people guess about 250 kilograms. That is very wrong. The digestive tract processes a staggering 30 tonnes of food in one human lifetime.

But what is food? Food is a deliciously complex array of particles often referred to as antigens. What we swallow includes food antigens – proteins, carbohydrates, sugars, fats, vitamins, phytonutrients, antioxidants, salts and minerals. It also includes genetic material from plants and animals and hormones from animals.

But there are also a multitude of living organisms on food, including viruses, bacteria, yeasts and parasites. Plus the bits of dead and broken-down bacteria, yeast and viruses. On top of this, we swallow a vast array of chemicals or food additives, called xenobiotics. These are not natural food products. They are foreign or manufactured chemical substances like drugs, pesticides, colourings, humectants, emulsifiers, flavourings and preservatives. There are thousands of chemicals that are used to make our drugs, cosmetics and processed or packaged foods.

The stunningly complex system of gut defences has evolved specifically to handle this massive chemical and microorganism load. Scientists probably stopped thinking of the gut as anything more than a digestive organ because the process of digestion and absorption is spectacularly complex enough. But, as anybody who has ever had food poisoning will attest, food can be dangerous to your health.

All too often the pleasure centres in our brain overrule our gut feelings. They can drive you, without any rational thought, to approach a local street vendor who is stirring a delicious-smelling pot of extra-spicy curry with a charred bamboo stick. You take a sniff. The food is heavily seasoned with spices to hide the smell of rotten meat and hydrogen sulphide gas being discharged by a toxic mix of *Salmonella typhi*, *Giardia* and *Vibrio cholerae* swimming in the lukewarm sauce. The poor, stick-thin, parasite-infested man hands you the cardboard bowl of curry, complete with a free serving of faeces that are caked onto his hands from a lifetime of using his bare hands to wipe away the residue smeared on his buttocks after repeated episodes of chronic diarrhoea. He has never been versed in food hygiene. He doesn't know that you shouldn't serve food if you have diarrhoea. He hasn't the foggiest idea what a formed stool looks like anyway, because he has never had one. He serves your curry on a bed of saffron rice that has been sitting out on his food cart since yesterday. It's had plenty of time to brew up a nasty batch of *Bacillus cereus*, a potent vomit-inducing bacterial toxin.

A sudden wave of revulsion washes over you. Your gut is saying, 'Please, no, something is wrong.' But you've had a couple of beers, you've been surfing, you're hungry and relaxed and you want to experience this different culture. Also, your bad Western gut bacteria are craving fat and sugars. The sensible, life-preserving message from your gut, which is now screaming, 'Don't eat that, you idiot!' is lost in the orgy of pleasurable sensations coming from the delicious-smelling food.

The gut goes quiet. It's in lockdown. It's too busy to keep warning you. It's preparing every available defence to face the onslaught of lethal bugs and toxins you are about to swallow.

You eat. You experience a satisfying sense of fullness from the saturated fats, a sugar rush from the carbohydrates in the rice, a tingle from the capsaicin in the chilli, and a spreading warmth from the curry powder.

The rest of your holiday is spent in grievous abdominal cramps. Your bum fires ring-scorching diarrhoea into the toilet bowl with enough power to blow a hole in the vitreous china. Your face strains over the bathtub as you spew bile-stained vomitus, like lava erupting from Mount Vesuvius. You call your best mate, who just happens to be a gastroenterologist. 'Froomesy, I swear I just chucked up the left lobe of my liver! I think I'm gonna die! What do I do?'

This is a true story. I received this call one night from a friend who was just two days into his honeymoon in Bali. After he was discharged from hospital, I asked him if he had felt any warning signals from his gut before the food touched his lips. He smiled and shook his head. 'Mate, how did you know? My bowels started cramping on me before the guy even handed me the bowl.' I knew because I know that the gut is wired into our brains. 'But I still ate it anyway!' He didn't listen to his gut.

The interplay between the food we eat, the digestive juices and gut hormones we secrete and the mass of metabolic bacteria that live in the gut has taken 2000 years to understand properly. We have finally acknowledged that the gut does a lot more than just digest and absorb food. In fact, this turns out to be the least of what it does. It is more concerned with protecting us from food than absorbing nutrients from it.

The next time you go out for a meal, stop and take a hard look at the food you are about to consume. Ask yourself this question: does this food look natural and healthy for my gut? Give it a moment. In that time, your gut brain will take in the information and form an impression. It will send a message back to the brain – a gut reaction – to convince the brain to react in a health-conscious way to the plate of food it is faced with. That will give you a good feeling or a bad feeling about the health and safety of that meal. I strongly encourage you to do this exercise. It will surprise you.

This is sometimes called 'mindfulness eating' but it's really gutfulness eating, because it's not your mind that's thinking about the potential threat on the plate, it's the gut. The brain is supposed to do the gut's bidding.

The reason the gastrointestinal tract is so vast is because it has developed a complex set of physical and biochemical systems to manage this multifaceted load of natural and manufactured compounds every time we eat. The gut is tightly linked to the brain through a complex gut-brain nervous axis, whose function is to let the brain know about good food sources and bad threats from our environment. The gut is directing the brain to act in ways that increase our survival.

# Chapter 11

## Where did gut bacteria come from?

By far the most strategically important of all the gut defences is the gut bacteria, collectively known as microbiota.

But where did these bacteria come from in the first place? Life on Earth has flourished since the first primordial meteors crashed into our fragile planet almost 3.9 billion years ago. Many scientists believe that those meteors carried and deposited ancient interstellar travellers, otherwise known as bacteria.[10]

According to this theory of evolution, those microbes gradually seeded our planet with organic material and inexorably changed the once-hostile environment to one that could sustain life.[11] In this scenario, bacteria are the biological engines that originally brought about and continue to shape all life on Earth.

This theory has many supporters, especially since we have discovered bacteria that have evolved to thrive in the most hostile environments on Earth. These superbugs are called extremophilic bacteria. *Dunaliella* algae live in caves in Chile's Atacama Desert – the driest place on the planet. *Aquifex* bacteria thrive in the hot springs of Yellowstone National Park at temperatures of 96 °C, close to boiling point. *Thermoccus* lives next to hydrothermal volcanic vents at the bottom of the ocean near New Guinea. Strange bugs like halophilic bacteria enjoy concentrations of salt that are ten times higher than sea water in the salt-lake beds of California. And psychrophilic bacteria live in frigid water below the polar ice. Other bugs are resistant to radiation, and some can even survive inside solid rock.[12]

Scientists believe that these rugged bacteria have found ways to survive space travel and exist all over the universe. Solar radiation winds blow bacteria-laden interstellar dust into planets, and microorganisms travel through space protected inside asteroids, meteorites and comets that crash into planets.

Researchers from India and Britain have found clusters of bacterial organisms thriving in air samples over 40 kilometres above the surface of the Earth, right at the edge of space. This is far beyond the reach of planetary microbes. And some

---

[10] Napier W, 2011, 'Exchange of biomaterial between planetary systems', *Journal of Cosmology*, vol. 16, pp. 6616-6642; Nicholson WL, 2009, 'Ancient micronauts: interplanetary transport of microbes by cosmic impacts', *Trends in Microbiology*, vol. 17, no. 6, pp. 243ol. 1

[11] Line MA, 2007, 'Panspermia in the context of the timing of the origin of life and microbial phylogeny', *International Journal of Astrobiology*, vol. 6, no. 3, pp. 249-254.

[12] Rampelotto PH, 2010, 'Resistance of microorganisms to extreme environmental conditions and its contribution to astrobiology', *Sustainability*, vol. 2, no. 6, pp. 16026, pp. Rothschild LJ & Mancinelli RL, 2001, 'Life in extreme environments', *Nature*, vol. 409, pp. 10921. 409

microbes have the ability to hibernate for millions of years, which would allow enough time for an interplanetary voyage almost anywhere in the universe.[13]

In 2001, researchers claim to have found extraterrestrial bacteria inside crystals of a meteorite that was estimated to be more than 4.5 billion years old. The bacteria had DNA unlike any on Earth and it survived even when the meteorite sample was sterilised at high temperatures and washed with alcohol.[14]

About 1 mg of dust from the Itokawa asteroid is being sent to Australia for Professor Trevor Ireland of the Australian National University to study. He is excited because these kinds of asteroids contain 'all sorts of organic molecules, and so may be seeds for the origin of life'.

If bacteria can survive space travel and are capable of making monumental changes to an entire planet, isn't it reasonable to take the bacteria that reside in our gut seriously?

Our modern-day bacteria are certainly the descendants of those interstellar microbes. They continue to shape our health and we continue to leverage their enormous genetic library to evolve our comparatively young human species. Yet medical practitioners continue to ignore the essential contributions of those bacteria to our health. We do so at our peril.

[13] Wickramasinghe C, 2010, 'Bacterial morphologies supporting cometary panspermia: a reappraisal', *International Journal of Astrobiology*, vol. 10, no. 1, pp. 25-30.

[14] Davies PCW, 2012, 'Footprints of alien technology', *Acta Astronautica*, vol. 73, pp 250-57.

# Chapter 12

# Are bacteria more evolved than humans?

We regard ourselves as the masters of our universe. We are undisputedly the most highly evolved species on the planet. We have developed complex brains and have a greater capacity to think, socialise and invent than any other life form. Yet, despite our advanced evolutionary state, we have been present on our planet for an archaeological heartbeat compared to the billions of years that bacteria have been co-evolving and shaping life on Earth.

Bacteria are the oldest living organisms on Earth. They have been here for billions of years and yet, for all that evolutionary time, bacteria have remained the same single-celled microscopic organisms. If Darwin's theory of natural selection is correct, why have bacteria not evolved into walking, thinking, self-aware organisms like us? Why have they remained in an evolutionary status quo? Could it be that bacteria are already so highly evolved that they will survive for eternity? If so, could bacteria already have a robust, innate intelligence that we are oblivious to simply because they are microscopic?

To dismiss bacteria as simple, unimportant, unicellular-organisms is monumentally naive. Their ancient structure has served them well, allowing them to survive mass extinction events, space travel and every hostile climate that this planet has to offer. What a perfect design for a terraforming life engine.

Bacteria may only consist of a single cell with a single piece of DNA to house their genes, but they have sophisticated genetic, manufacturing and communication systems that will ensure they survive well beyond the era of humans.

Bacteria have developed resistance to every antibiotic ever invented. No amount of money or Nobel Prize-winning microbiologists can invent drugs that kill bacteria as quickly as those same bacteria develop drug resistance. So who are the true geniuses?

The first step in the development of antibiotic resistance is a genetic change in a single bacterium. There are two ways this can happen. The bacterium can undergo a spontaneous genetic mutation. Many antibiotics work by inactivating an essential bacterial protein. Genetic changes can alter that protein so the target of the antibiotic is gone but the protein still functions. Other mutations can prevent the antibiotic from binding to the bacteria or prevent it from inactivating the target protein. Spontaneous genetic change might lead to increased production of the antibiotic's target protein so that the antibiotic can't inactivate them all. Alternatively, the bacterium may produce an antibiotic-inactivating enzyme.

The second way that a bacterium can gain resistance to an antibiotic is for an existing antibiotic-resistant gene to transfer from one bacterium to another.

Bacteria have small circular DNA structures called plasmids that allow for the exchange of genes from one bacterium to another. Microbiologist John Turnidge says they literally borrow their resistance genes from neighbouring bugs. 'They're the original life forms almost, so for thousands of millions of years they've had a chance to work out ways to survive and one of those is to borrow genes from other bacteria to survive.'

# Chapter 13

## So you think you're human

It's reasonable to assume that most of us think of ourselves as intrinsically human. But just how much of that is really true? If a spaceship full of inquisitive aliens were to visit Earth, what would they think of us? If these alien travellers put a human in their cell analyser machine, the conclusions they would draw about us might be very far removed from what you and I might imagine.

From the results of cell analysis, they would conclude that a human being is made up of around ten trillion human eukaryotic cells and 100 trillion bacterial cells. Which means that, cell for cell, we are only 10% human and 90% bacterial.

What about our DNA? We are the most complex and highly evolved creatures on the planet, and this is due to our intricate genetic structure. The human genome is composed of a vast array of different genes that encode our unique and supreme structure and function. Well, it turns out that humans contain about 20,000 genes, but humans also contain over 2,000,000 bacterial genes. Gene for gene, we are only 1% human and 99% bacterial. Our alien visitors might quite rightly conclude that we humans are a walking framework or carrier animal for our bacterial masters.

Why is it that a worm has 20,000 genes, a tree has 45,000, the flowering Japonica has 1.2 million, yet we humans have only 20,000? In part, we have managed with relatively few genes because of the vast sea of bacterial genes in our gut that we leverage to perform many complex functions for us. Our combined genome consists of more than 2.5 million genes. This composite human genome and gut bacterial microbiome is now referred to as the 'metagenome' and medical researchers regard humans as 'super-organisms'.

It strikes me as no coincidence that people who claim to have been abducted by aliens all report a similar experience – anal probing. I used to laugh at this but now it seems perfectly logical. Inside the anus are the bacteria that make up 99% of our genes!

Within each human body, the bacterial microbiota and 'host' human cells form a complex ecosystem that performs a multitude of interactive biological processes in a synergistic balance.

We have co-evolved this mutually beneficial balance with our resident gut bacteria from the moment we crawled out of the primordial ooze two-and-a-half million years ago. The essential relationship between humans and our gut bacteria has been honed to an evolutionary perfection that benefits us both. This mutual evolution began from the time humans split off the evolutionary tree from a common ancestor that gave rise to three hominid pathways of evolution: humans, chimpanzees and bonobos. Studying the DNA sequences in humans suggests that we diverged from chimpanzees and bonobos five to seven million years ago.[15] We still all share similar gut bacterial phyla that were passed on to us from our common ancestors, but we humans have had almost seven million years of specific human-bacterial evolution that has gone into perfecting exactly the right balance of resident gut bacteria to maximise our, and their, survival.

---

[15] Prüfer K et al, 2012, 'The bonobo genome compared with the chimpanzee and human genomes', *Nature*, vol. 486, no. 7404, pp. 527-531.

# Chapter 14

# The big bang of birth

Our traditional thinking was that a newborn baby acquires its first microbiome with the 'big bang' of childbirth. The passage through the maternal vagina literally smothers the baby in a sea of microflora that grow over the baby to protect it. The truth is that our relationship with bacteria begins well before birth.

We have always considered the uterus to be a sterile and protective environment that shields the vulnerable foetus from the evils of bacteria and germs. Like so many medical concepts, this has turned out to be wrong.

The microbiota of the birth canal is around 80% *Lactobacillus*. But research has found that a newborn's gut microbiota is significantly more diverse and contains a range of other bacteria. So where does the foetus get these bacteria from? The developing foetus is exposed to a number of maternal bacteria that circulate in the amniotic fluid of the womb. Because the foetus swallows amniotic fluid, all these bacteria get into the gut and arm the foetus with its first film of gut bacteria well before birth. The placenta also has a diverse colony of microbes. The placental microbiota metabolise vitamins just like gut bacteria do, which is better for a newborn who is about to get their nutrition from milk rather than umbilical cord blood.

This wholescale colonising of the newborn infant with bacteria is one of the most important requirements to sustain life. A baby must rapidly envelop itself with a protective biofilm of bacteria to survive the myriad of dangerous infections that exist outside the safety of the uterus. Newborns need gut bacteria to digest milk. They also need to train their fledgling immune system to recognise and defend them against bad bacteria and learn not to attack good bacteria.

Babies are still exposed to a microbial 'big bang' of sorts during birth, when they collect good bugs from their mother's vaginal canal that rapidly colonise and enrich the existing foetal microbes. Babies delivered by caesarean section tend to have lower bacterial cell counts in faecal samples. Other microbial hits come from both their mother and father's skin and saliva and from breastmilk.

Breastmilk is as much about assisting with bacterial colonisation of the gut as it is about nourishment. We have known for a long time about the protective effect of antibodies in breastmilk. These antibodies help the newborn fight off infections that the mother's gut has detected in the environment she has delivered her baby into. But the true complexity of breastmilk composition is even more interesting. Breastmilk has its own microbiome too!

Every time the newborn sucks at the breast, they are getting a top-up of more good bacteria to help colonise and protect and extract nutrients for their gut. And, just like the gut microbiome, every mother has a unique composition of breastmilk bacteria. Every woman has different genetics, different dietary patterns and lives in a slightly different environment. She naturally acquires and passes on to her infant the bacteria that are best adapted to her environment.[16]

Unlike other mammals, scientists have recently discovered that human mothers produce a staggering 200 different complex sugars in their breastmilk. Most of these sugars can't be digested or absorbed by the baby. They pass undigested to the small bowel and colon. All these sugars are there for one reason only – to provide nourishment for the baby's developing gut microbiome. This complex sugar mixture in breastmilk selectively promotes growth of the most important neonatal gut bacteria. These bacteria perform two essential functions for the neonate. Firstly, they digest some of the components of breast milk, allowing the infant to absorb these milk nutrients. Secondly, they prepare the infant gut for future solid food digestion. Bacterial colonisation allows the infant gut to switch to a diet that is not exclusively based on milk before the actual change in their diet takes place. This is a huge advantage for both bacteria and infants.[17]

From infancy onwards, our diet has a powerful influence on the make-up of our gut microbiota. As an infant grows, we introduce it to solid foods that are rich in natural carbohydrates. These feed beneficial strains of good bacteria, allowing the developing gut microbiota to acquire a broad range of different probiotic bacteria. This process is called increasing biological diversity and it is very important. Our gut needs many different strains of bacteria to obtain maximum health benefits.

These initial bacterial colonisers of the gut are replaced by a broader range of probiotic bugs by about the age of one. These bugs are specific to the infant and different from those found in their mother and siblings. A developing toddler's gut microbiome matures toward an adult-like microbiome at around the age of two-and-a-half. At the same time, the gut immune system learns to differentiate between the resident probiotic bacteria and disease-causing pathogens. By the time the child reaches adulthood, a relatively stable community has been achieved. The gut microbiome signatures of adults are as individual and different as fingerprints or retinal patterns.[18]

It turns out that your gut bacteria even effect how clever you are. There are specific microbial strains of 'smart bacteria' that when colonising your gut from infancy can make you smarter than other kids. Cognitive testing of 89 two-year-old kids using the Mullen Scales of Early Learning, which tests how advanced their brains are in terms of gross motor, fine motor, visual reception, expressive

[16] Hunt K et al, 2011, 'Characterization of the diversity and temporal stability of bacterial communities in human milk', *PLoS One*, 6(6), e21313.

[17] Marcobal A et al, 2011, 'Bacteroides in the infant gut consume milk oligosaccharides via mucus-utilization pathways. cell host microbe', *Cell Host Microbe*, vol. 10, no. 5, pp. 507-514.

[18] Koenig J et al, 2011, 'Succession of microbial consortia in the developing infant gut microbiome', *Proceedings of the National Academy of Sciences of the United States of America*, vol. 108, supplement 1, pp. 4578-4585.

language and receptive language skills, ranked the infants according to how clever they were.

Faecal microbial analysis of these infants showed that the really brainy infants all had the same gut bacterial clusters and that they were quite different in composition to the gut microbes of the less intelligent infants. This led the researchers to conclude that certain gut bacteria enhance infant brain development and function. In other words, the microbial composition of your infant gut can determine your cognitive ability – i.e. how clever they are.[18.2]

One day we might have a way of enhancing all human intelligence by breeding a clever gut microbiome in our infants!

---

[18.2] Alexander L et al. 2018, 'Infant Gut Microbiome Associated With Cognitive Development'. *Biological Psychiatry*, 83:148-152.

# Chapter 15

## Faecal microbial transplant

There are only so many ways you can change the microbial make-up of your gut. A high-fibre diet and probiotics have been the most easily accessible methods so far. But most people struggle to achieve significant results with either of them because both these interventions require long-term adherence. Understandably, most people are not brilliant at sticking to diets or taking capsules forever.

Studies show that changes in your diet can alter your gut bacteria within just a few days. So the minute you hark back to your bad old eating habits so does your gut bacteria.[19]

Probiotic supplements don't change your underlying resident microbial population. At best they just help out. Probiotics lose their temporary benefits and disappear completely from the gut within two weeks of stopping them.

These shortcomings have led us to explore more effective ways of changing the gut microbiota. The most promising strategy thus far is called faecal transplant (FMT). FMT has turned out to be so effective it has become the 'end game' of transforming a sick gut microbiome back into a healthy one.

It's based on the simple principal of transferring a suspension of gut microbes contained in a stool from a healthy person to a sick person, whose illness is related to gut bacterial infection or dysbiosis.

But, before we talk more, you should know that this form of gut microbial reloading is not part of a regular program to reboot your gut bacteria. FMT is still undergoing extensive research and as such it is reserved for those who fail to respond to all the standard measures discussed in this book, and it is only for those who have correctly diagnosed *Clostridium difficile* infection, ulcerative colitis, Crohn's disease or irritable bowel syndrome with gut bacterial dysbiosis, and have not responded to standard treatments. Even some of these indications are hotly debated in the medical world.

FMT should never be done unsupervised by a doctor at home because of the potential for bad outcomes like transfer of infections, obesity or mood changes from inadequate screening of donors or improper handling of transplant material. In the end, most people will not need it. But for those in need of it, FMT is sometimes a miraculous treatment.

The concept of swapping faecal microbes between humans has been part of our medical culture for centuries. Animals all do it by nibbling at each other's poo from time to time. We humans are the only animals that fail to do this.

It all started in fourth-century China, when a bold Chinese healer named Ge Hong became the first person ever recorded to start giving a suspension of faeces from healthy persons to those affected by severe diarrhoea. There have been many reports since of using the faecal suspension referred to as 'yellow soup' for a variety of gut problems. The vets have been using FMT for decades to treat animals with diarrhoea. But it wasn't until 1958 that the first report of using faecal transplant enemas for humans infected with *Clostridium difficile*, that causes a nasty form of colitis, hit the medical literature.

In 2017, what we currently do is start with a great poo donor. Donors for FMT must meet strict health criteria and pass a battery of blood and stool tests, termed the Amsterdam protocol, to ensure they cannot pass on any untoward health problems or infections to the recipient. Some people use relatives because their similar genetic profiles may assist the new bacteria taking up residence in the recipient but the catch is the related donor may share the same type of disease susceptibility, whether genetic or environmental, as the recipient. Most cases now use non-related, properly screened donor banks.

Next we prepare the transplant. The donor has to deliver a fresh stool sample, one that has been passed on to the lab within four hours of collecting it. The processing lab mixes 50g stool with 200ml of sterile saline water and blends it until smooth. This watery poo slurry is passed through a coarse filter to remove large particles and the remainder is then drawn up into syringes. If it is to be frozen, a cryoprotectant is added before freezing at -70 degree C.

Once an FMT has reached room temperature it must be used within six hours. FMTs are usually administered up the bum as an enema but can also be given via a colonoscopy to the far end of the large bowel or given down into the small intestine by gastroscopy or nasojejunal tube. These days various labs are investing in poo capsules and freeze-dried FMTs but these are yet to be properly studied for efficacy.

What's in an FMT? At present, we assume it's all just good probiotic bacteria and that is what gives FMT all its therapeutic power, but research has shown there is a lot more to it.

FMTs contain a variety of viruses, called bacteriophages. These little viruses live in the bowel and protect us from infection by killing off pathogenic bacteria and they are so good at it that they are used in the food industry to prevent contamination of food by such nasties as *Salmonella, ETEColi* and *Staphylococcus*. There are also a variety of antimicrobial proteins in the FMT slurry called defensins that also attack bad gut bacteria and help prevent dysbiosis. FMTs are brimming with short-chain fatty acids butyrate, propionate and acetate. These nutrients provide a fuel source for gut cells, promote normal intestinal permeability by inducing production of tight junction components and send calming signals to the intestinal immune system. Finally, micro RNA particles have also been found in stools. mRNAs are gene signal proteins or messengers that can turn off inflammation in the gut. There are many ways and FMT might actually be working and this may be why fresh and frozen FMTs still work best.

FMT has really excelled in the treatment of *Clostridium difficile*. Once your gut microbiome has been decimated by antibiotics, this resistant bacteria *C diff* can take over the gut and produce a toxin that damages the lining of the colon so badly it can be lethal. We believe FMT works in *C difficile* infection by restoring the microbial richness of the gut microbiome. This allows reconstitution of your natural bacterial defences against *C diff*. And it works stunningly well. The global mean cure rate of antibiotic resistant *C Diff* infection with FMT is 91%.[19]

Is it the new bacteria from the donor that are responsible? The answer is yes. Bacterial gene sequencing studies show that recipient gut microbiome closely resembles that of the donor at two weeks after FMT and furthermore it has been shown to persist in some cases as long as two years.[20]

FMT is showing great promise in chronic inflammatory bowel disease. The latest multi-centre, randomised controlled study was conducted in Australia with 42 patients with moderately severe ulcerative colitis. After eight weeks 44% of patients had all their symptoms of colitis disappear and had stopped taking steroid drugs entirely. This is better than the most potent immunosuppressant drugs available that induce remission in only 33%. [21]

A meta analysis done on the effect of FMT in Crohn's disease from 134 studies and 88 patients has shown a clinical remission rate of 50.5% with FMTs.

In IBD, the best responses were with multiple donor infusions and multiple infusions. [22]

While there is less data on FMT in irritable bowel syndrome, some work has shown significant response rates. A small study of 13 patients with chronic IBS showed FMT resolved or improved symptoms in 70% of patients. With improvements in 'abdominal pain (72%), bowel habit (69%), bloating (50%) and flatus (42%). FMT also resulted in improved quality of life (46%)'. [23]

A patient of mine, let's call her Sophie whom I treated with FMT, wrote about her experience of changing her microbiome with FMT below. It illustrates where we are at with FMT very well.

> 'My name is Sophie, and I am 47 years old. I have had 'bad tummy problems', eczema and other allergy symptoms since age nine which gradually worsened over the years and I became quite sick in 2007/8, when all my symptoms multiplied and became very severe. This is despite numerous conventional (strong cortisone and other creams, U/V therapy) and natural treatments (diets, herbal medicines, homeopathy, etc). I drew the line at internal cortisone and immuno-

[19] Colleen R. Kelly et al. Fecal Microbiota Transplant for Treatment of *Clostridium difficile* Infection in Immunocompromised Patients. Am J Gastroenterol, 2014.133; 1065-1071.

[20] Ranjit Kumar et al. Identification of donor microbe species that colonize and persist long term in the recipient after fecal transplant for recurrent *Clostridium diff* Biofilms and Microbiomes (2017) 3:12.

[21] Paramsothy S et al. Multidonor intensive faecal microbiota transplantation for active ulcerative colitis. The Lancet 2017;389 (10075);1218-1228.

[22] Paramsothy S et al. Faecal microbial transplant for inflammatory bowel disease: A systematic review and meta-analysis. J Crohns Colitis May 9, 2017.

[23] Brandt L et al. Long-Term Follow-Up of Colonoscopic Fecal Microbiota Transplant for Recurrent *Clostridium difficile* Infection. Am J Gastro 2012;107:1079-1087.

suppressive drugs, considering them not addressing the cause of the problem. From 2009 I started seeing an integrative medicine GP and we found out eventually that I have multiple food sensitivities, multiple chemical sensitivities (notably all scents including perfumes, essential oils, etc); candida overgrowth and leaky gut/intestinal dysbiosis. This explained why diets excluding single or just a few food items never worked for me as I was still reacting to other items, and why herbal medicines, juicing, concentrated food supplements and fermented foods never helped me; in fact, they only made me worse and this has puzzled many a naturopath. However, finding the cause did not lead to any permanent solution. I still had a lot of symptoms on a daily basis despite major changes to my life. Things were still up and down. Fatigue was such a big issue; I stopped working as a naturopath (also because of disillusionment) and had to reduce my work hours as a physiotherapist drastically.

At the end of 2014 I decided to have an FMT – faecal microbial transplant. It's been the single item that has made the most consistent and most global results to date. I have been told I will improve over several years with regular top-ups. (Following my initial five FMTs in December 2014, I have had a total of seven top-ups in the past 12 months.) It is still experimental at this stage for IBS and there are a lot of unknowns. I have noticed improvements in many of my symptoms including sleep, memory/cognition, moods, (calmer/able to handle stress better), energy and motivation, skin, gut and digestion, hair, joint and muscle pains, weakness, immune system, sinuses etc. I have also been able to stop or reduce some of my medications/supplements that I couldn't do without before. The list is not exhaustive and the improvements are not always immediate. I started studying Masters part-time this year – I would not have been able to cope with it if not for the FMTs. However, I am not there yet, ('it's a long, long road...' ) as my favourite lyrics go). Recently, I had a severe exacerbation of all my symptoms in spring – traditionally a bad time for me. Thankfully an FMT enema top-up, whilst not returning my health to pre-spring levels, again significantly improved my symptoms. It was amazing to see the rash on my body fade away within a few days, retreating back to its 'normal' areas. The FMT is the only thing I've found that makes a big difference.'

The point often missed in all the hype about FMT is that sometimes it doesn't work. While hundreds of studies have proven it safe and free of any serious side effects, the key to unlocking the best ways of using FMT and of improving its effectiveness is still unknown. Until then, many people will get great benefit from it but many will see nothing at all.

At this point in time, the application of FMT for everything else such as autism, multiple sclerosis, diabetes, obesity, Parkinson's disease, lupus, psoriasis, fibromyalgia, depression and rheumatoid arthritis is still in the realm of case reports and theory, but studies are already in the pipeline in many of these disorders and we await the results with great anticipation.

# Chapter 16

# What's in your poo?

Once thought to be nothing more than rejected foodstuffs, poo has turned out to be a fascinating window into the wildlife sanctuary that resides in our bowels. Poo is literally bursting with live (and dead) viruses, bacteria, microorganisms, yeast and parasites. It also contains a swag of antibodies, hormones, neurochemicals, proteins, short-chain fatty acids and DNA-like particles, called messenger RNA, that tell our gut cells how to behave.

Medical science has focused its microscope squarely on colonic gut bacteria as potentially the most influential of all the bugs living it up in the bowel. This has spawned an industry that encapsulates certain stool probiotic species to use as treatments for illnesses that involve the gut. It has even gone as far as creating person-to-person faecal microbial transplants. The healthy bacterial mass contained in the FMT is then administered as an enema into the bowel of the unhealthy person, creating a new and healthy gut microbiota that will heal them of their ailment.

But, given all the other goodies in the faecal transplant mix, it just may be that FMT works because of the unique combination of both bacterial and the ingredients in the stool mix. This might help explain why FMT is so much more effective than probiotics. After all, a faecal transplant is brimming with small molecules that have positive effects on the gut lining, gut nervous system and gut immune system such as short-chain fatty acids, chitins, antimicrobial proteins, defensins, beneficial viruses called bacteriophages and micro RNA particles. None of these compounds are found in probiotic capsules.

These days anyone can pay to have their poo zoo analysed. The problem is that not many doctors know how to interpret these results, and even fewer non-medical people understand what these results might actually tell you. I'm going to give you the basics, but be warned this field is changing rapidly. What we know is still very limited, given the vastness of the human gut microbiome.

So far we have an initial but basic picture of what might be a healthy state from a gut microbial perspective. Scientists have used DNA mapping techniques to investigate the genetic composition of the gut microbiome of people from six different nationalities. They took bacterial DNA from thousands of people and compared them to genetic libraries generated by the American National Institutes of Health's Human Microbiome Project and the European Meta HIT consortium.

From these analyses, we know that a normal human gut zoo consists of around one quadrillion viruses, 100 trillion bacteria, one trillion archaea, and a bucketload of yeasts, protozoa and fungi. Currently, when we analyse and refer to the gut microbiota, we are talking almost exclusively about the 100 trillion bacteria.

When you have your stool gut microbiome tested, the gut bacterial microbiota consists of around $10^9$-$10^{12}$ colony-forming units of bacteria per gram of stool. Anaerobic bacteria account for the bulk of the microbiota, outnumbering aerobic bacteria by 1000 to one. Of the anaerobic bacteria, at least 80% of the make-up of anaerobic bacteria appear to fall into one of three general patterns, called enterotypes. These enterotypes are *Bacteroides*, which predominate when your diet is rich in protein and fats, *Prevotella*, which predominate with a high carbohydrate diet, and *Ruminococcus*, which tend to be favoured by a diet high in refined sugars. But not surprisingly, in the Western population Ruminococcus was the most common.

More recent and larger studies have found that the human gut microbiota contains at least 1800 different genera of bacteria, with over 16,000 different phylotypes at the species level and another 36,000 different phylotypes at the bacterial strain level. The human intestinal microbiota turns out to have a much greater diversity than any microbiologist or microscopic zookeeper imagined in their wildest dreams.

Before we look more closely at the microbiome, it might help to remember some high school biology, in particular, the hierarchy of biological classification. This classification system is science's way of defining groups of biological creatures based on their evolutionary similarities. It includes seven divisions, starting with the kingdoms: animalia, fungi, plantae, chromista, protozoa, archaea and bacteria. Each sub-classification that follows divides organisms into smaller and more specific groups. In descending order, these are kingdom, phylum, class, order, family, genus and species.

As far as gut bacteria go, the vast majority belong to just four bacterial phyla. So the first result you are likely to get from an analysis of your poo zoo is the breakdown of the phyla that your gut bugs belong to.

| Bacterial phyla | |
|---|---|
| Firmicutes | 40-60% |
| Bacteroidetes | 10-30% |
| Proteobacteria | 8% |
| Actinobacteria | 3% |
| Verrucomicrobia | 2% |
| Archaea | 1% |
| Fusobacteria | <1.0% |
| Others | <0.5% |

You generally want your gut bacterial spread to be within the ballpark percentages described above. The lab will then break down these big groups into the smallest groups they can, which is usually only to the genus level.

| Phylum | Class | Genus |
|---|---|---|
| Firmicutes | Bacilli | *Lactobacillus*<br>*Klebsiella*<br>*Enterococcus*<br>*Citrobacter*<br>*Streptococcus* |
| | Clostridia | *Clostridium*<br>*Blautia*<br>*Ruminococcus*<br>*Faecalibacterium* |
| | Erysipelotrichia | |
| | Negativicutes | |
| Bacteroidetes | Flavobacteriia | *Flavobacterium* |
| | Bacteroidetes | *Bacteroides*<br>*Prevotella* |
| Proteobacteria | Gammaproteobacteria | *Enterobacter*<br>*Escherichia*<br>*Thalassospira* |
| | Alphaproteobacteria | *Oxalobacter* |
| | Betaproteobacteria | *Desulfovibrio* |
| | Delta/Epsilon | |
| Actinobacteria | Coriobacteriaceae | *Collinsella*<br>*Bifidobacterium* |
| Verrucomicrobia | Verrucomicrobiae | *Akkermansia* |
| Archaea | Methanobacteria | *Methanobrevibacter* |

The names of the bacteria at the genus level are often familiar, as some of them are used as probiotics. The really interesting thing is what species are in our gut and what they really do. We are only just beginning to understand what a good gut microbiome should look like, what genes each subspecies contains and what metabolic products these genes code for.

The myriad of other minor taxonomic divisions are hugely diverse in different individuals, which means your individual gut microbiota are unique to you. Besides these 'snapshot' analyses of intestinal microbiota composition, other long-term surveys have followed both the overall composition and that of individual people for periods ranging from several months to two years. These longitudinal studies suggested that the composition of intestinal microbiota in adults doesn't change drastically within these periods.[24]

---

[24] Manimozhiyan A et al, 'Enterotypes of the human gut microbiome', *Nature*, vol. 473, no. 7346, pp. 174-180.

# Chapter 17

## What do probiotics do?

Until recently, science and medicine hadn't the foggiest idea that bacteria might actually be helpful, let alone essential to human health. This attitude was spawned by the lifesaving power of antibiotics to cure infections. And what causes infections? Bacteria! The idea that microbes might be essential for good health has mostly been ridiculed. Nobody doubts that pathogenic bacteria taking up residence in parts of the body leads to infection. However, the fact is that the vast majority of bacteria living both outside and inside our bodies have turned out to be essential for our health. Without them, we would not function or be able to defend ourselves.

Try to think of the relationship between humans and probiotic gut bacteria as one where humans provide a warm, safe, nutrient-rich home for bacteria to thrive, and in return the bacteria do everything they can to ensure our health and survival.

Good bacteria really do protect us from infection. Our probiotic gut microbes encase us in a microscopic protective suit. These great little bacteria secure themselves in the nutrient-rich mucus layer of the gut and proliferate until they reach the largest possible sustainable population. Once we have a gut grandstand packed to bursting with good bacteria, they suck up every last micronutrient our diet can provide and starve out bad bacteria.

The competition for nutrients between good and bad bugs in the gut is fierce, but it doesn't stop there. Good bacteria also provide significant competition for invading bacteria by blocking their ability to attach to the gut mucus lining. Bad bugs can't get a grip – they get swept away down the toilet with the stools. Good bacteria also produce their own mini antibiotic molecules that attack and destroy pathogenic bacteria that try to invade the gut. The front line of defence against infection from bad bugs is our own probiotic gut bacteria.

Good gut bacteria also help build and maintain a healthy gut lining. They do this by talking to the enterocytes and stimulating them to produce strong mucus, the protective gut antibody sIgA, and the tight junction proteins. They secrete amino acids and short-chain fatty acids that control and regulate gut movement and maintain the gut lining and mucus.

Gut bacteria produce hundreds of essential chemicals. Of particular interest is the ability of certain good bacteria to manufacture three essential amino acids: tryptophan, phenylalanine and tyrosine. These critical nutrients provide the building blocks for the neurotransmitters dopamine, serotonin and melatonin. In the gut, these neurotransmitters regulate movement, secretion, muscle contraction and pain sensation. However, in the brain, dopamine is one of the key mediators of happiness and pleasure, serotonin induces relaxation and calm, and melatonin regulates sleep. If you've ever wondered why you constantly feel grumpy, anxious and can't sleep, it's because of your bad gut bacteria. Having the right balance of good bacteria in your gut keeps you happy, calm and ensures a good night's sleep.

The bacteria in the colon play integral roles in nutrient absorption. It is the action of colonic bacteria that leads to the formation and absorption of vitamins like biotin, vitamin B12, thiamine, riboflavin and vitamin K. The bacteria also produce the gases – carbon dioxide, hydrogen and methane – that make up flatus.

*Escherichia coli* (*E. coli*) is another important species that makes essential amino acids and vitamins as well as the coenzyme CoQ10. CoQ10 is a vitamin-like substance that is present in most human cells and is a key component of the energy production pathway. This pathway generates energy in the form of an energy-loaded molecule called ATP. Ninety-five per cent of the human body's energy is generated this way. ATP can carry its energy to anywhere in the body.

Gut bacteria also protect you against cancer. Many reports describe gut bacteria like *Lactobacillus* and *Bifidobacterium* binding to a variety of food-borne carcinogens including the heterocyclic amines formed during cooking of meat, the fungal toxin Aflatoxin B1 and the food contaminant AF2.[25] These handy little probiotic bacteria actively bind and destroy a variety of carcinogens we don't even realise we've eaten. They also have a very useful enzyme system called glycoside hydrolysis. This bacterial enzyme can generate a number of potential anti-carcinogenic and anti-mutagenic substances like flavonoids, such as quercetin.[26]

If food-borne carcinogens that we eat manage to get past our probiotic gut bacteria, the gut lining and the liver will try to inactivate them. Scientists have shown that the probiotic *Bifidobacterium longum* and the prebiotic inulin can inhibit precancerous growths in rodents by nearly 80%.[27] So probiotic bacteria really do their stuff.

[25] Daniluk Y, 2012, 'Probiotics, the new approach for cancer prevention and or potentialization of anti-cancer treatment', *Journal of Clinical & Experimental Oncology*, vol. 1, no. 2.

[26] Hullar M et al, 2014, 'Gut microbes, diet and cancer', *Cancer Treatment Research*, vol. 159, pp. 377-399.

[27] Rowland IR et al, 1998, 'Effect of *Bifidobacterium longum* and inulin on gut bacterial metabolism and carcinogen-induced aberrant crypt foci in rats', *Carcinogenesis*, vol. 19, no. 2, pp. 281-285.

# Chapter 18

# Common gut bugs

A basic understanding of the general role of some of the more common bacteria that reside in the gut helps a little when browsing thorough one's stool microbiome results. This is a field that is rapidly changing as analysis of bacterial genes and metabolic processes is now taking off. Here's an introduction.

We'll start with Firmicutes – one of the most common microbes in the human gut. Firmicutes are great digesters of animal fats, and fats are a rich source of energy. As hunter-gatherers, a gut full of Firmicutes helped us lay down fat stores after eating big meals of meat. This allowed us to live through harsh winters when food was scarce. Life ain't so tough these days. Foods high in fat and sugar are stacked on every supermarket shelf. And an oversupply of Firmicutes in the gut is associated with a higher risk of obesity.

Some Firmicutes are notorious pathogens and cause diseases such as botulism and anthrax, but the vast majority are both completely harmless and necessary for normal digestion. Outside the human gut microbiome, some Firmicutes species can actually ferment beer and wine and turn milk into yoghurt.

A very important genus of Firmicutes is *Lactobacillus*. These bacteria populate the entire length of our digestive tracts and play a major role in commercially-produced probiotics. They protect against infectious germs and help other probiotic microbes thrive in the gut. They are also the dominant subtype of bacteria found in the vagina, where they protect against vaginal and urinary infections, and populate the guts of vaginally-delivered infants. They ferment sugars and oligosaccharides to produce lactic acid. This keeps the pH of the gut and vagina tract slightly acidic, which protects against yeasts and other pathogens.

Babies who start out with fewer lactobacilli are more likely to develop allergies later in life, and in turn giving *Lactobacillus* supplements to infants at high risk for allergies and asthma may prevent those conditions from developing. Lactobacilli are not always good bacteria, though. When too many grow in our mouths, the acid they produce can cause tooth decay. Both vitamin B6 and biotin promote lactobacilli growth.

Another important member of the Firmicutes phylum is *Clostridium*. Some *Clostridium* species are nasty. These bugs can cause botulism and enterocolitis. But most are beneficial species that make up part of our healthy flora. Like any probiotic bacteria, they can cause issues if they become too plentiful. A retrospective study of 60 patients with intestinal dysbiosis found that the prevalence of *Clostridium* species in the intestinal tract was related to the symptom of constipation. The higher the *Clostridium* count, the more likely it was that the patient had complained of constipation. People with chronic diarrhoea might benefit from more *Clostridium,* but those with constipation need less.

The most important member of the Actinobacteria phylum is *Bifidobacterium.* Bifidobacteria are among the most well-studied organisms in the human colon, as they are believed to play an important role in lifelong health. They ferment sugars and produce lactic and acetic acid. They are abundant in the gut of infants and may protect the gut from inflammation. Because of their usefulness, many species are sold as over-the-counter probiotics, though there is limited data on their efficacy. Regularly consuming yoghurt with live cultures has been shown to maintain higher levels of bifidobacteria .

Both *Lactobacillus* and *Bifidobacterium* reinforce intestinal permeability, prevent the attachment of pathogenic bacteria, assist the breakdown of plant-based carbohydrates and increase the nutrients that we can absorb from certain foods.

The other kingpin of the Actinobacterium phylum is *Collinsella* (previously called eubacterium). These bacteria are some of the biggest producers of the important short-chain fatty acid butyrate, which is essential for maintenance of healthy gut mucus. They also assist in the digestion and absorption of dietary fats and help bile acids to be reabsorbed and returned to the liver for continued use. Low levels of *Collinsella* in the gut microbiome are associated with diarrhoea from fat malabsorption.

The phylum Bacteroidetes are the most prominent gut microbes in most of the world's population, expect for people who eat a lot of meat. Bacteroidetes are thought to help protect against obesity because they do not digest fat well. The first settlers of Europe had to digest fat to give them enough energy to survive the brutal Ice Age winters. People with fewer Bacteroidetes and more fat-digesting Firmicutes became dominant. That is why meat-eating Westerners have more Firmicutes than Bacteroides even today.

Bacteroides are highly efficient at breakdown of plant-based foods. They thrive on fruit and vegetables and can release many of the vitamins, minerals and energy from carbohydrates that our human digestive systems cannot do alone. They provide a rich source of short-chain fatty acids that are both anti-inflammatory and provide the predominant energy source for the cells of the gastrointestinal system.

*Prevotella* are turning out to be a troublesome member of the Bacteroidetes phylum. While some species are useful members of the healthy microbiome of the mouth and vagina, others have been implicated in anaerobic infections of the airways and lungs like aspiration pneumonia, lung abscess, pulmonary empyema, chronic otitis media and sinusitis. They have been isolated from tooth abscesses, bites, urinary tract infections, brain abscesses and osteomyelitis. One species of *Prevotella, P. copri,* has been implicated as a possible trigger for the development of rheumatoid arthritis. *Prevotella* are seen more often in the bowels of people who eat a high, simple-carbohydrate diet.

A recent discovery in the phylum Verrucomicrobia is the bacteria *Akkermansia*. *A. muciniphilia*, the only known species in this genus, has been found to be a very important probiotic. It is thought to be protective against obesity, diabetes, and inflammation. *Akkermansia* appear to be highly sensitive to feeding times – their levels rise as they feast on the mucin secreted by cells in the gut wall during fasting. Even a fasting period of less than 24 hours has been shown to increase overall gut diversity. Eating foods like garlic, onion and bananas feeds the *Akkermansia* in your gut. More work is needed on these potentially important bacteria.

One of the most well-studied members of the phylum Proteobacteria is *E. coli*. These guys are the good *E. coli* bacteria (not the toxin-producing ones that cause outbreaks of gastroenteritis) that assist in the digestion of carbohydrates and nutrient absorption. *E. coli* coliforms are important intestinal microorganisms that are responsible for the synthesis of essential amino acids and vitamins. They also produce glucosamine, which is an essential component of cartilage for good joint function.[28]

In summary, medicine is finally coming to realise what Hippocrates knew 2000 years ago. The gut is intimately connected to health and disease. As long as your gut and its bacteria are balanced and healthy, it will go about its business without bothering you. But what happens if your gut is unbalanced?

---

[28] Gruber J & Kennedy BK, 2017, 'Microbiome and Longevity: Gut microbes send signals to host mitochondria, *Cell*, vol. 169, no. 7, pp. 1168–1169.

# Section 2

# When gut bacteria go wrong

# Chapter 19

# Leaky gut

Bear with me. We are about to delve into how your intestinal microbes cause disease, so this section might get a little technical. Put simply, we are going to discuss how your gut microbiome becomes messed up (gut dysbiosis), how your gut barrier becomes too permeable (leaky gut) and why this helps diseases to develop.

For some reason, the term 'leaky gut' seriously irks most doctors. Say it out loud and they scoff and turn away in disgust. This might be because the term itself doesn't sound clever – it has no Latin roots and has a decidedly non-medical feel – so they decide it must be a total load of rubbish. Leaky gut is not rubbish. Fifty thousand medical journal articles have confirmed it.

So what is leaky gut? As we discussed earlier, leaky gut occurs when our gut lining becomes too permeable. This means it lets the wrong kind of things get from the intestine into our body. The gut lining is really just a barrier between our gut bacteria and what we eat. It's a single layer of intestinal cells (enterocytes) that are chained together by arms called tight junctions. These are the gate-keepers of the gut. The gut barrier decides which molecules are nutrients, and can be allowed into our bodies, and which molecules are not and are locked out. It makes millions of these decisions every day.

Most food nutrients pass directly into and across the cells lining the gut. However, there are also tiny gaps between the gut cells that let some molecules in. These gaps are controlled by the tight junctions. Only a few select substances are allowed to pass across the gut barrier. Since our bodies can only use nutrients that are broken down to tiny single molecules, any particle larger than a single molecule is shut out. This is because it is either bacteria, a toxin or a bit of food that is too large for us to use.

When this barrier becomes leaky, a flood of bad molecules can pass through the gut lining and into our bodies. This is not good. These substances will be identified as foreign by both our gut's immune system and our body's immune system and attacked. This sets up inflammation in the gut and the body and may even trigger autoimmune disease.

So how do we know when things are starting to go wrong? One way is to measure gut permeability. The intestinal permeability test (IPT) is a simple test that is often used in clinical studies. The test works by dissolving two sugars, mannitol and lactulose, in a cup of water and drinking it. You collect your urine for several hours afterwards and the laboratory measures how much of each sugar there is in your pee.

Mannitol is a small monosaccharide that's readily absorbed through the enterocytes. Some of the mannitol is always excreted in urine. Lactulose is a larger disaccharide that is too big to be absorbed and shouldn't appear in urine. The only way lactulose can get through is when you have leaky gut. The more lactulose there is your urine, the worse your intestinal permeability defect is.

Many things can damage the gut barrier and make the gut too leaky, including toxins and metabolites produced by dysbiotic bacteria. More worrisome is that our Western diet does exactly the same thing. The food we eat not only contains natural food molecules that alter gut permeability, such as gluten, capsicum and cayenne, but at least 300 different processed food extracts and chemical food additives go into all the packaged, refined, processed and canned foods we consume in abundance. These modern foods induce abnormal gut permeability either by forcing tight junctions open too wide or by damaging the proteins that they are constructed and breaking them down.[29] Either way, leaky gut is the result. Of course, the amazingly adaptable machine that is our body can handle temporary abnormal changes in gut permeability. The problem occurs when permeability is chronically abnormal.

| Causes of leaky gut | |
|---|---|
| Gut dysbiosis | Overgrowth of dysbiotic bacteria with undergrowth of probiotics |
| Diet | Gluten, capsicum, cayenne, food chemicals, alcohol |
| Medication | Steroids, antibiotics, NSAIDs, aspirin, chemotherapy |
| Infection | Cholera, salmonella, yeast, parasites |
| Stress | Elevated cortisol releasing peptide, adrenaline, noradrenaline |
| Hormone deficiency | Thyroid, oestrogen, progesterone, testosterone |
| Physical | Stroke, brain injury, surgery, trauma, burns |

And what about alcohol? While we are not certain how much alcohol affects gut permeability, studies show that if you expose intestinal lining cells to a solution containing 5% alcohol it disrupts the proteins of the tight junctions and increases permeability. Therefore, alcohol consumption can potentially cause

---

[29]   Ulluwishewa D et al. Regulation of tight junction permeability by intestinal bacteria and dietary components. The Journal of Nutrition. 2011;141:769-776.

leaky gut, and the significance of this effect is probably related to the volume of alcohol consumed.[30]

How does stress cause leaky gut? Stress causes increased blood flow to skeletal muscles and decreased blood flow to the gut. Good blood flow to the gut is critical for the delivery of oxygen and other nutrients required to maintain barrier function. When exposure to stress is chronic, it leads to persistently high levels of the stress hormone corticotropin-releasing factor (CRF). CRF is thought to cause histamine release from special white blood cells in the intestine called mast cells, and histamine disrupts tight junctions and increases gut permeability.

In response to a breakdown in the gut barrier, the intestinal cells and immune cells release inflammatory chemicals (cytokines) to fight off the intestinal food antigens and bacterial toxins that slip past the protective gut lining. But these cytokines also have an inflammatory effect on the gut. They sensitise the gut nerve endings, driving you crazy with sensations of discomfort and pain.

So now you know some of the reasons for all the fuss about leaky gut!

---

[30]  Wang Y et al, 2014, 'Effects of alcohol on intestinal epithelial barrier permeability and expression of tight junction-associated proteins', *Molecular Medicine Reports*, vol. 9, no. 6, pp. 2352 Rep6.

# Chapter 20

# Gut dysbiosis

We have learned that the human body contains more than 10 times more bacterial cells than human cells, and over 100 times more bacterial genes than human genes. The mass of microorganisms that make up the human gut microbiota of a modern Western human weighs around two kilograms. It is as metabolically active as the body's powerhouse, the liver, and is now considered so important by most experts that it is classified as a separate human tissue.

Your gut bugs have an overwhelming impact on your health. Since most of these microbes are impossible to grow in a lab using current methods, it was not until advanced DNA sequencing technology became available that we began to identify them. These techniques have revealed that the bugs that call our bowel home are so important that we practically need to create an entirely new subspecialty in medicine for them.

It turns out that abnormalities of the gut microbiome are implicated in chronic IBS, autoimmune diseases like diabetes, rheumatoid arthritis, systemic lupus erythematosus (SLE), multiple sclerosis (MS), chronic fatigue, obesity and some cancers. Since some of the microbes in our body can modify the production of neurotransmitters found in the brain, we are finding the gut bacteria also have a role in sleep, mood, depression, anxiety and other neurochemical imbalances.

The real issue for Western societies is that our diets are skewed towards encouraging the overgrowth of bad or dysbiotic bacteria and discouraging the growth of good or probiotic bacteria. Dysbiotic bacteria are non-health-promoting bacteria that do not confer one iota of health benefit to their human host. Mainstream medicine has finally recognised the concept of dysbiotic bacteria and has christened them with the unpronounceable name 'facultative pathobionts'. We'll stick to dysbiotic bacteria.

Dysbiotic bacteria are different to the pathogenic bacteria that cause a specific, sudden-onset illness. Dysbiotic bacteria starve us of nutrients by reducing probiotic levels, and slowly poison us from within by producing toxins and noxious gases. They thrive on the Western diet that is high in refined sugars, overcooked saturated fat, carbohydrates from white flour and processed seed oils, and low in fibre.

The lack of dietary fibre in our Western diet actively discourages growth of health-promoting probiotic bacteria. Tip into the mix the fact that germ-phobic Westerners continually ingest a probiotic-killing blend of pesticides, disinfectants and antibiotic residues and you have a perfect recipe for a weak microbiome. Specifically, a microbiome that is lacking in lots of different types of probiotics (biodiversity), low in probiotic mass and dominated by the wrong types of bacteria. This sets us up for illness.

Modern Western societies are awash with heart disease, obesity, diabetes, strokes, autoimmune disease and cancers. Most of these health problems were virtually unknown in hunter-gatherer societies, where the diet was moderate in saturated fat, omega 3 fats and protein, while high in fibre and completely devoid of sugars (apart from a bit of honey) and grains. The gut microbiome of people living in developing countries is far more biodiverse and weighs between four and six kilograms. That's two to three times the mass of the average Western gut microbiota.

A healthy gut microbiome is one that is balanced. That means it is predominantly made up of probiotic bacteria. All too often, dysbiotic bacteria overrun the probiotic bacteria. In essence, there is a constant turf war going on in the bowel between the dysbiotics and the probiotics.

| Conditions that favour dysbiotic bacteria and lead to leaky gut | |
|---|---|
| Western diet | Sugar, grains, gluten, white flour, fructose, saturated fats, seed oils |
| Treated water | Most drinking water is chemically treated with chlorine and fluoride |
| Chemicals | Pesticides, disinfectants, antiseptics, preservatives, colouring |
| Antibiotics | Damage probiotic gut bacteria |
| Drugs | Non-steroidal anti-inflammatory drugs (NSAIDS), cytotoxic drugs, chemotherapy, radiation |
| Gut infections | Viral, bacterial, parasite, yeasts |
| Stress | Stress hormones alter gut microbiome |

The effects of gut dysbiosis are threefold. Firstly, we miss out on the benefits, anti-inflammatory effects and micronutrients that probiotic bacteria offer us. Secondly, we are exposed to a multitude of toxic bacterial by-products and inflammatory effects of dysbiotic bacteria. Thirdly, the production of fatty acids, which are fuel for the gut wall cells, is reduced and the function of the gut barrier becomes impaired. The transfer of toxic by-products of bacterial sugar fermentation across the gut wall occurs and these chemicals end up in our bloodstream. Not only do we feel unwell, but the mechanism thought to underlie autoimmune diseases has begun.

A dysbiotic microbiome and a Western diet are the main drivers of gut wall damage and increased permeability.

# Chapter 21

## Why do we have bad gut bugs?

So why is our microbiome out of balance? We need look no further than our evolution to find the answer. *Homo habilis* was our earliest ancestor and fossils of this primate date back some 2.3 million years. *Homo habilis*, like all the hominids that followed, were hunter-gatherers, which means they ate wild meat and fish, berries, seeds, vegetables and roots. Humans – and our gut bacteria – have spent nearly two-and-a-half million years adapting to this diet.

Until about 10,000 years ago, there were no farmers, no domestic animals and no crops. Evidence suggests that humans probably consumed almost no grains at all. There were no antibiotics, pesticides, food chemicals, colourings, and the nutrient quality of soil (and therefore plants and animals) was rich. It has been estimated that the soil was as much as 10 to 20 times more nutrient-dense than it is today.

The person who published the first work on this was Dr Boyd Eaton. He estimates that *Homo sapiens* left behind their hunter-gatherer ways to raise animals and grow crops around 7000 to 10,000 years ago. It wasn't until about 5000 years ago that agriculture had taken over on all continents. This massive change in lifestyle has been termed the Neolithic revolution. Our diet changed to crops, grains, fruits, wheat flour, cow's milk and meats from domesticated cows, sheep, goats and pigs. Quite a shock for the gut microbiome.

In the modern era, we have added even bigger drivers of gut microbial change. The first was antibiotics. Penicillin was discovered by accident by the bacteriologist Alexander Fleming in 1928. After a trip to Scotland, Fleming returned to his laboratory to examine his petri dishes. He had been growing culture plates of *Staphylococcus*. *Staphylococcus* is a bacterial pathogen that causes skin infections and blood infections. Much to Fleming's annoyance, some of his petri dishes had grown mouldy over the break. Instead of chucking them out, he looked at them and noticed that the plates with mould on them had no *Staphylococcus*. That mould was *Penicillium notatum*. The mould killed *Staphylococcus!*

It took another 13 years for Australian Professor Howard Florey to develop the technology to isolate and extract penicillin from the mould. He needed 2000 litres of mould culture fluid to extract enough penicillin to treat a single patient. Only then was penicillin's potential to kill bacterial infections acknowledged by the medical profession. Mass-scale fermentation processes were then developed to produce antibiotics on a commercial scale. Bacterial infections that had once maimed and killed millions of people were curable at last. Antibiotics became the most prescribed medication in history.

This is when gut probiotic bacteria started to come under serious fire. In 2015, figures released by the UK's National Institute for Health Care and Excellence confirmed that over 4,000,000 prescriptions for antibiotics were written in the UK alone. Not surprisingly, they also believed that one in three antibiotic prescriptions were unnecessary. Even today, we reach for antibiotics at the slightest hint of illness.

The second big driver of gut dysbiosis was the wholesale addition of sugar and high-fructose corn syrup to almost all processed foods. Humans are hopelessly susceptible to and captivated by sugar. Our cerebral pleasure centres have no defence against its hypnotic sweetness. We are so enamoured of it that the processing of sugar has become a billion-dollar industry. A magical pinch of sucrose or fructose makes absolutely anything taste delicious, and people pay handsomely for it.

In 1953, Kellogg's released their best breakfast cereal yet: Honey Smacks. These beauties contained 56% by weight refined sugars. They were stuffed with a diabolical mix of sucrose, fructose and dextrose. The other 44% of the Honey Smacks was made up of processed wheat. By 1957, high-fructose corn syrup had replaced sugar in soft drinks. It is the most potent sweetener on the planet and people just can't get enough of it. The world now produces 180 million tonnes of sugar per annum, and sugar and corn syrup are like fertiliser for dysbiotic gut bacteria.

The third big driver of gut dysbiosis happened 66 years ago with the founding of McDonald's in San Bernardino, California. The McDonald's brothers quickly discovered that fried burger meat, deep-fried potato chips and sugar-laden milkshakes got people so hooked that by 1948 the fast-food chain was unstoppable. McDonald's now has over 35,000 outlets operating worldwide. This is dysbiosis food.

It is fascinating to observe that in 1950, just two years after McDonalds spread throughout the USA, one of the first references to the concept of an 'irritable bowel' appeared in the *Rocky Mountain Medical Journal*. The term was used to categorise patients who developed chronic symptoms of diarrhoea, abdominal pain and constipation, but where no physical cause could be found. As a result, most early theories about IBS were that is was a mental disorder.[31] It has taken almost 60 years for us to fully appreciate the role of gut bacteria in IBS. Sugar, antibiotics and fast food are destroying our gut microbiome.

In practice, our microbiome tends to get messed up by one of three events: antibiotics, a bout of gastroenteritis or a time of high stress. Many people can pinpoint the onset of their gut problems to one of these events. The rest are a product of poor diet and lifestyle.

---

[31] Brown PW, 1950, 'The irritable bowel syndrome', *Rocky Mountain Medical Journal*, vol. 47, no. 5, pp. 343-346.

Effects of overgrowth of bad bacteria can be severe. For example, sulphate-reducing bacteria (SRB) are bacteria that can reduce sulphate to hydrogen sulfide gas ($H_2S$). Effectively, these bugs 'breathe' sulphate instead of oxygen. $H_2S$ plays a major role in making gut nerves hypersensitive and slows down bowel movement.

*Streptococcus* and *Enterococcus* are aerobic bacteria that produce lactic acid from glucose. They are potent producers of two types of lactic acid: L-lactate and D-lactate. Both these forms of lactic acid are readily absorbed across the gut into our bodies. By making the colon too acidic, these lactates kill good probiotic bacteria like *Bifidobacterium* and *Bacteroides*. L-lactate is metabolised in the liver and high levels of this may indicate bowel overgrowth with *Streptococcus*. But D-lactate is the problem. Our livers cannot metabolise it, so it accumulates in human tissues. This is a particular problem for our energy factories, which are called mitochondria. D-lactate inhibits energy production by mitochondria which means less energy for your body and more fatigue. We can measure D-lactate in the bloodstream to assess for this. High levels of *Streptococcus* and *Enterococcus* growing in the bowel significantly and positively correlate with cognitive dysfunction such as nervousness, memory loss, forgetfulness, confusion and the mind going blank.

The other side of gut bacterial dysbiosis is an undergrowth of beneficial gut bacteria. This is both a general lack of volume and species of good gut bugs as well as fewer specific individual probiotic bacteria. Without good numbers of these health-inducing probiotic bacteria we lose the nutrients they make for us and the protection they offer against infections. We are in a weakened state both nutritionally and immune defensively. Secondly, without good gut bacteria we lose the ability to tolerate our own gut bacteria. When this happens, we run the gauntlet of chronic over-stimulation of the gut immune system. This is believed to be a pivotal trigger for IBS, food allergies and autoimmune diseases.

There is a delicate balance of good versus bad bacteria living in our gut. When the gut microbiome becomes unbalanced and an unhealthy diet predominates, the gut generates significant inflammation, pain, maldigestion, malabsorption and IBS. An imbalance in the intestinal microbiome may be associated with bowel inflammation and may also trigger food allergies and autoimmune diseases.[32]

---

[32] Marteau P, 2009, 'Bacterial flora in inflammatory bowel disease', *Digestive Diseases*, vol. 27, pp. 99-103; Lepage P, 2012, 'A metagenomic insight into our gut's microbiome', *Gut*, vol. 62, no. 1, pp. 146-158.

# Chapter 22

## Gut bacteria and irritable bowel syndrome

IBS has always been considered a functional gut syndrome because there is nothing structurally wrong with the gut and there is no identifiable disease process associated with it. IBS sufferers have been viewed with scepticism, as if they are malingerers or their problem exists only in their heads. But thanks to advances in DNA technology, scientists have confirmed that IBS is caused by an imbalance in the gut bacteria.

The characteristic hallmarks of IBS, which include excessive gas production, abnormal motility, gut nerve hypersensitivity and low-grade inflammation, arise from a noxious combination of dysbiosis and low-level gut irritation from poor diet and leaky gut. The microbial imbalance in the gut creates a constant stream of gut immune activation and gut nerve overstimulation. In addition, the gases and chemicals liberated by dysbiotic bacteria have been shown to alter gut motility and impair digestion. This drives even worse symptoms from food that is not absorbed properly.

Studies have consistently shown that, compared with healthy controls, people with constipation-predominant IBS (IBS-C) have gut dysbiosis characterised by an increased population of sulphate-reducing bacteria (SRB) and Clostridial species and a deficiency of *Bacteroides*.[33]

When you attempt to correct the dysbiosis with a change in diet, probiotics or faecal microbial transplant (FMT), things can change. A study of 45 patients with chronic IBS-C treated patients with one colonoscopic FMT followed by a series of faecal enema infusions from donors who had a very regular bowel habit. They found that after FMT 89% of patients were able to resume regular defecation, and had a significant reduction in bloating and abdominal pain immediately after the procedure. Nine to 12 months later, 60% of them were still going to the toilet daily, without laxative use.[34]

Diarrhoea-predominant IBS (IBS-D) often happens after the gut microbiome has been damaged by an attack of gastroenteritis or a course of antibiotics. People with IBS-D have a significant gut dysbiosis, which is marked by a reduction in biodiversity of the faecal microbiota. They also have overgrowth of *Ruminococcus torques* and some *Bacteroides*, and reductions in *Clostridium*

---

[33] Chassard C et al, 2012, 'Functional dysbiosis within the gut microbiota of patients with constipated-irritable bowel syndrome', *Alimentary Pharmacology and Therapeutics*, vol. 35, no. 7, pp. 828-838.

[34] Andrews P et al, 1995, 'Bacteriotherapy for chronic constipation – a long term follow-up', *Gastroenterology*, vol. 108, no. 4, A563.

*thermosuccinogenes*, various species of *Lactobacillus* and *Bifidobacterium*.[35] Changing the gut microbiome with FMT can also reverse IBS-D.[36]

The medical literature is finally starting to accept this.

> '...medicos can quite reasonably speculate that the microbial intestinal dysbiosis that exists in D-IBS patients may play a role in causing IBS. Certainly, we know that immune chemicals released in the gut have been shown to activate sensory afferent neurons involved in visceral pain and enteric nervous system responses, and may be linked to abnormal gut secretions and gut motor activity.'[37]

This was written in 2009. It's official! But forgive your doctor. They will only be aware of this if they have read the literature and they cannot always be across every new development that occurs in medicine. You could spend seven days a week reading medical journals and still be behind.

The effects of dysbiosis on the gut are largely due to the action of multiple noxious chemicals released by overgrowth of bad bacteria. One of the most annoying things dysbiotic bacteria do is ferment carbohydrates to produce gases. Some gases smell offensive and are toxic to the gut, while others are more inert. The main problem for the patient is bloating, offensive flatulence and gaseous distension of the belly. These gases can upset the pH of the gut as well as gut motility, causing constipation or diarrhoea, and they can irritate gut nerve endings, causing pain. Colonic fermentation can be measured by the colonic pH and changes in pH correlate well with IBS.[38]

Let's take a look at what the typical IBS patient experiences when they try to solve the problem and how they fare with a traditional medical approach. All IBS patients tread a common path. It usually begins with a bout of gastroenteritis, traveller's diarrhoea, a stressful event or a course of antibiotics. You get over the initial illness but you're never quite the same again. You experience recurring bouts of bloating, gas and abdominal discomfort. Your gut makes more noises than before, you may have a little nausea or heartburn and your bowel habits have changed into a mix of diarrhoea, constipation and normal. You may not be too fussed at first. You tell yourself it will probably settle down soon.

But it continues, so you try a few home remedies and over-the-counter medications from your local pharmacist, like antacids, charcoal and

---

[35] Lyra A et al, 2009, 'Diarrhoea-predominant irritable bowel syndrome distinguishable by 16S rRNA gene phylotype quantification', *World Journal of Gastroenterology*, vol. 15, no. 47, pp. 5936-5945.

[36] Borody TJ et al, 1989, 'Bowel flora alteration: a potential cure for inflammatory bowel disease and irritable bowel syndrome?', *Medical Journal of Australia*, vol. 150, no. 10, p. 604.

[37] Piche T et al, 2009, 'Impaired intestinal barrier integrity in the colon of patients with irritable bowel syndrome: involvement of soluble mediators', *Gut*, vol. 58, no. 2, pp. 196-201.

[38] Ringel-Kulka T et al, 2015, 'Altered colonic bacterial fermentation as a potential pathophysiological factor in irritable bowel syndrome', *American Journal of Gastroenterology*, vol. 110, no. 9, pp. 1339-1346.

antispasmodics. For stomach pain, you try aspirin, paracetamol, ibuprofen or other non-steroidal anti-inflammatory (NSAIDS) pain relievers (the second most common over-the-counter medication sold today).

When these treatments don't work, you go to your doctor for a prescription to stop bowel cramps and too much acid, like Colofac and Buscopan, or strong acid-blocking drugs called proton pump inhibitors (PPIs). Then you discover that the most common side effects of antispasmodics are dry mouth, blurred vision and constipation. PPIs can cause headaches, diarrhoea and abdominal pain. For some people, the medications create more problems on top of the IBS symptoms. Wonderful!

Next you try to tackle your frustrating and unpleasant irregular bowel habit. For diarrhoea or loose bowel movements, you take a constipating agent like Imodium or Gastro-Stop. If you have constipation, you take a laxative or fibre supplement like Metamucil, Coloxyl with senna or Fybogel, or a stool softener like Movicol. These drugs don't seem to work either. If the constipation or diarrhoea continues, it's again off to your doctor for an even stronger laxative or constipating medication.

Somewhere along the way you realise that certain foods make your gut ache worse and you are afraid to eat them. You try a variety of diets suggested by your naturopath or dietician but none of them really help. In fact, now you seem to be developing sensitivities to even more foods. Your symptoms are getting so severe that you are reluctant to leave the house and, when you do, you have to know the location of every bathroom between your home and your destination. Congratulations, IBS now rules your life.

If your pain continues or gets stronger, your doctor may refer you to a surgeon to see if you need your gall bladder out. They've found nothing else to explain the doggedly persistent symptoms, and the medical profession believes you don't really need your gall bladder anyway. But unless you have gallstones, removing the gall bladder rarely results in any relief. And without it, you experience additional digestive symptoms because you now have a reduced inability to efficiently digest rich, fatty foods.

Since none of these over-the-counter medications, prescriptions, dietary changes or surgical solutions resolve your problem, it's off to the doctor again. By now they're probably tired of seeing someone that they don't really have the tools or knowledge to help, so they refer you to a gastroenterologist.

Gastroenterologists are specialists in the intestinal tract. They are trained to perform unique testing to rule out more serious conditions like inflammatory bowel disease, peptic ulcers, coeliac disease or cancer, and they are all excellent at that. You undergo a series of stool tests, colonoscopies, endoscopies, barium enemas, MRIs and CT scans. You are tested up this way and down that way, and your specialist reassures you that all the tests are negative and there's nothing seriously wrong with you. It's just an irritable bowel – a minor ailment – and everybody knows that you can live with that. Yet you still have all your symptoms and you know something is very wrong.

Do not despair. All of this is an essential part of the journey. A correct diagnosis is the only way you are going to get the correct treatment. After all, an IBS program is not going to fix Crohn's disease or bowel cancer. Being checked out properly by your doctor and your gastroenterologist first is absolutely essential.

You try to cope as well as you can, but the toxic effects of chronic bowel bacterial imbalance are taking a psychological toll on you. You're still anxious about your gut problems, you're having trouble sleeping and you are constantly fatigued and moody.

Continued visits to your doctor result in an unspoken, industry-wide red flag that your problems are due to stress. You don't need me to tell you how furious it makes you when this label is plastered across your medical file. You are prescribed an antidepressant or referred to counselling or a psychiatrist. 'So you have IBS,' your doctor says, and his eyes begin to glaze over. You can feel the interest in your problems evaporate as fast as a drop of sweat off a back of a dung beetle baking in the hot Sahara sun.

A practitioner telling you that this is all in your head is not only unfortunate, it is completely wrong. In my opinion, IBS sufferers are told far too often that their bowel problems are due to them being too emotional, too tense or over-anxious. That maybe they should just calm down, go home and feel better about feeling so bad. But who wouldn't be stressed by living with the unrelenting symptoms of chronic IBS? By the time people come to see me, many of them have indeed developed secondary psychological symptoms of anxiety, stress, poor sleep, fatigue and even depression as a direct result of the chronic gut bacterial dysbiosis that now runs their lives.

It's an unfortunate journey. There are no positive results, your quality of life continues to deteriorate, you might be taking antidepressants that you don't need and you are wasting a lot of money.

Could your doctor be right? Is there no cure? Must you learn to live with IBS? I believe the answer to that question is definitely 'no'. The answer is simple. We have to go back to the basic biochemistry, physiology and microbiology of the gut to find the answers. Once you treat a dysbiotic gut microbiome, IBS can be cured. The case below proves my point.

A 49-year-old woman came to see with terrible IBS-C that she had been suffering for over 20 years. After having children, it had only gotten worse. She was only opening her bowels once every two weeks, despite taking up to 40 laxative tablets every night. She was constantly bloated, craving sweet foods, physically sluggish, fatigued, had gained weight and suffered stomach distension almost every afternoon that made her look seven months pregnant. All of this was making her anxious and depressed. She had seen many doctors and naturopaths and even a psychiatrist. None of the probiotics, diets, medications or laxative regimes she had been given had made any real impact. She had practically given up, until she saw a program on TV about faecal transplant.

I treated her dysbiosis first to wipe out her unhealthy microbiota and followed this with a regime of faecal transplants from specially selected donors who had regular twice-daily bowel habits. Suddenly, things started to change. Within two weeks she was opening her bowels every three days and had reduced her nightly laxatives to 10. I added a daily probiotic blend and within four weeks she was opening her bowels every second day and taking no laxative tablets at all. Her bloating, anxiety and mood all lifted. She could not believe the response. After three months, her healthy regular bowel habit continued, she was laxative-free, and she had lost almost 10 kilograms. Her sugar cravings had stopped and she was eating a lot more fruits, salads and vegetables. When she came to my office, she couldn't stop smiling.

While pharmaceutical companies and great medical minds continue to research the complex neuroendocrine pathways of the gut in order to develop better drugs to treat IBS, the real solution is to correct the underlying gut microbial imbalance, repair the intestinal lining and restore normal digestive function. This approach is the key to helping an IBS sufferer regain their quality of life.

The personal journey, written by one of my patients below, is all too common in the world if IBS. But, in many people, changing the make-up of the gut microbiome can make a real difference.

My experience had a slow build; my hair was dying and my fingernails were breaking. After eating I would be curled up in ball with stomach pains that would last 30-90 mins or need to sleep for hours. I noticed that the cleaner I ate, the worse I got. Gluten free, dairy free, used coconut or nut product replacements, low FODMAP … but I continued to get worse. I needed to use the bathroom 10 times a day; it felt like I always needed to go and I was forever in pain.

My issues peaked at work. I am a firefighter. I work in an environment where I need to be well and ready to respond to any task within 90 secs and may not have access to a bathroom for many hours. I had started to make my own Acai bowls; this final morning I finished my delicious breakfast and within 20 mins I was on the change-room floor. I couldn't move. My partner had to come get me from work and drive me to the doctors.

The next few days were spent at home, taking 4-6 Imodium a day.

The next few weeks was everyone's standard story – seeing my local doctor, then being referred to a gastroenterologist, getting a gastroscopy and colonoscopy or 'top & tail' as its affectionately called, having stool and blood tests, and going back to the gastro only to be told 'you have IBS and we are 10 years off understanding the gut. Go see a dietician'.

The next few months were spent on elimination diets, food tests and multiple visits with my dietician. I was so sensitive that the only food I could have had to be safe on several diets for me to eat it. It had to be Low Failsafe diet, Low FODMAP, gluten free, dairy free, nut free, coconut free, no preservatives, no additives… I could only have blueberries and half a green banana for fruit. I could have six veggies and they had to be peeled, I could have salt but not pepper, I could have chicken but no skin, beef but it couldn't be aged, no pig of any type, fish but not canned. I could only have water for months on end as even peppermint tea's food chemical content was too high.

I was surviving but changing my diet was only a Band-Aid; it wasn't solving the problem.

I then saw a new gastroenterologist who was interested in the gut microbiome, Dr Froomes. I had to do more detailed stool tests but these showed I had no good gut bacteria at all and leaky gut with major food hypersensitivities. The plan of attack was his eight-week gut microbiome repair program, four phases of two weeks each. 1. Kill the bugs, 2. Repopulate with good bugs, 3. Seal the leaky gut, 4. Fix hypersensitivity. The first phase made me so sick that on the last day of taking the antibiotics I had to go home from work. I later found out I was in toxic shock from the bad bugs dying, which was a good sign. Things settled in the second stage.

But by the end of the program I was doing really great. I ate normally and likely too quickly as within six weeks I was sick again and had to do the program a second time, but needed to reintroduce food slowly at the end of it. This second attempt made me more sensitive. I also became histamine sensitive, I started having flushes, dizziness and had become so food chemical sensitive that I couldn't have slow-cooked meat with what I knew were safe ingredients. During these programs I dropped to 58 kgs (I'm 5'11) and struggled to consume more than 800 calories a day, with half of that being fail-safe potato chips (I had to check the packets for ingredients and the oil used to cook the potato).

My relationship with food had changed. I was scared of eating out as every meal or drink came with many questions, weird looks and the risk of feeling very ill after it. All I did was think about the food I couldn't eat. All day, every day, was food. I collected recipe book after recipe book and on really tough days I couldn't be around my work mates while they ate their meals. My social and home life was hugely affected; I became isolated and withdrawn. I could only eat if I had prepared meals in advance, every single meal. It got to a point where I'd make one batch of food and eat the same meal for lunch and dinner, days on end. I'd lost the passion I once had for being in the kitchen.

Dr Froomes explained that it was time for the last resort, a faecal microbial transplant (FMT). I had no alternative. I had five treatments over eight days, all from different donors with the first via a colonoscopy and the other four self-administered as enemas. It's not a choice you make lightly and it was beyond difficult to get my head around. It took months for me to be able to talk about it and I took time off work to do the transplants. The concept of what I was doing to myself was difficult … but I had to weigh up, do I continue to be miserable with no end in sight or potentially live a normal life, eating again, like everyone else…?

It's only now that I can really see how much the gut is connected to the brain. I can see now that I was down, I was in survival mode, my body image had been warped, my weight loss had become the normal and I struggled with the concept of normal weight. I struggled with every mouthful. Each bite had three worries attached to it; 1. Will this make me sick? 2. Will this make me fat? 3. Will this feed the bad bacteria we've tried so hard to beat and undo all of the work we've done? Every forkful carried guilt and worry.

I now am nine months post FMT. I am better. I have a normal life. I know the foods that might give me a little tummy ache now and then and I can tolerate more and more items as time goes by. I was so well that I took a trip to Europe and ate and drank my way through each country. I had high anxiety levels before going. What's Europe without food? I did great! Everything tasted wonderful and I was able to slowly eat worry free.

My food guilt has reduced, my self-image has been restored and my motivation for enjoying food and cooking has returned. I am in the best place I have been for years. I have energy again; I can order something from a restaurant menu without asking a dozen questions, I am finally happy again. Having the FMTs gave me my life back. It was a last resort but it was the right choice.

# Chapter 23

# Gut bacteria and small intestinal bacterial overgrowth

If you get bloating, stomach aches and cramps, nausea and distension of the belly within 30 minutes of a meal it's highly likely that the problem is dysbiosis or bacterial overgrowth in the small intestine. Thirty minutes is way too early for the meal to arrive in the colon, so the symptoms must be coming from higher up.

Small intestinal bacterial overgrowth (SIBO) is a critical disturbance in gut bacteria caused by bacteria that normally reside in the colon creeping up and taking over the small intestine. SIBO is often overlooked and poorly understood by practitioners. Unlike the colon, which enjoys $10^{14}$ or more bacteria per ml, the small intestine can only handle a certain load of microbes. When you have more than $10^{14}$ bacteria per ml in the small intestine, you can have SIBO. This calculation can be performed on small intestinal fluid by suctioning it up during a gastroscopy.

The other way to make the diagnosis is by a glucose breath test. Our intestine is adept at absorbing glucose because it is the primary fuel for the brain and muscle cells. If you drink a cup of glucose mixed in water there should be no increase in hydrogen or methane in your breath. The only way breath hydrogen or methane can increase after drinking glucose is if there are masses of bacteria in the small intestine that are sucking up the glucose and producing excess gas. These gases are absorbed into the bloodstream and breathed out by the lungs.

What do these microbes do in the small intestine? They do what they do best – ferment your undigested food like crazy and produce a host of irritant substances. They also produce methane and lactic acids, both of which alter the motility of the small intestine, giving you pain, distension and diarrhoea or constipation. Finally, the excess bacteria are seen as a threat by the gut immune system and immune activation can result. The end result of all this is gas, bloating and pain.

But it can get even worse. Excess bacteria in the small intestine can destroy your bile salts, prevent the absorption of fats, cause malabsorption of the fat-soluble vitamins A, D, E and K, deactivate vitamin B12 absorption, and consume dietary sugars and proteins and deprive our bodies of them. This is called small bowel malabsorption and it can result in nutritional deficiencies.

Studies show that SIBO is a significant problem.[39] It is present in 30-46% of people with IBS. The worst sugar for promoting SIBO is fructose. Small intestine bacteria go mad for it. Many bacteria utilise fructose to make a type of fructose

---

[39] Lacy B et al. The treatment of irritable bowel syndrome. Therapeutic advances in gastroenterology 2009; 2(4); pp. 221-38.

chain that helps them stick onto the lining of the small intestine. This is how they promote their own bacterial overgrowth.

SIBO can occur in the proximal small intestine, mid small intestine or distal small intestine and the timing of symptoms produced reflect this. The quicker you feel crook after your meal, the higher up in your small bowel the bacterial overgrowth is likely to be.

The traditional approach to managing SIBO has been to kill off the overgrowth with antibiotics, which does give symptomatic relief to many people. The problem with SIBO is that it often returns. This leads to recurrent courses of antibiotics, the risk of inducing antibiotic-resistant gut bugs and severe dysbiosis of the large bowel. It can become a never-ending cycle.

Any program aimed at eradicating SIBO has to include dietary changes to restrict the sugars that encourage the bacterial overgrowth and improve the motility of the small bowel, and a short course of antibiotics or herbal antiseptics to lower the bacterial load at the start.

Although some people experience worse symptoms when taking probiotics as a result of increasing the bacterial mass in their small bowel, studies have shown a benefit from taking one of three probiotic strains – *Lactobacillus casei, L. johnsonii* or *Bacillus clausii*.[40] All were effective in relieving the symptoms of SIBO and/or returning the glucose or lactulose breath tests to normal. Making changes to the composition of the microbiota in the small bowel can also improve motility and symptoms of IBS.

---

[40] Aragon G et al. Probiotic therapy for irritable bowel syndrome. Gastroenterology and hepatology. 2010:6(1); 39-44. Zhong C et al. Probiotics for Preventing and Treating Small Intestinal Bacterial Overgrowth: A Meta-Analysis and Systematic Review of Current Evidence. J Clin Gastroenterol. 2017 Apr; 51(4):300-311.

# Chapter 24

# Gut bacteria and autoimmune disease

Fifty years ago there were very few known autoimmune diseases. Now there are over 80 separate, clearly identified autoimmune diseases including type 1 diabetes, coeliac disease, SLE, Sjögren's syndrome, rheumatoid arthritis, Crohn's disease, ulcerative colitis, MS, Parkinson's disease, autoimmune hepatitis, primary biliary cirrhosis, mixed connective tissue disease and Hashimoto's thyroiditis, just to name a few. Autoimmune diseases affect one in 20 Australians and these diseases are increasing at an alarming rate. Their impact is global, with over 100 million people afflicted. The bad news is that they have no cure. They are treated with lifelong immunosuppressive drugs.

Chronic autoimmune diseases are the by-product of your immune system recognising bits of yourself (self-antigens) as foreign, which can lead to inflammation and destruction of your own specific tissues and organs by your own immune system.

The current classical theory of autoimmunity involves two hits. The first hit is to be born with a genetic predisposition to an autoimmune disease. Autoimmune disease inheritance is complicated, with lots of different genes controlling various aspects of susceptibility to autoimmunity. All autoimmune diseases have clear associations with a group of genes called human leukocyte antigen (HLA) genes. HLA genes have direct involvement in the immune system function.

The second hit is a change in gut bacteria. The way that gut bacteria trigger autoimmune diseases is simple. We are all made of similar stuff, as it turns out. Bacteria all have a cell wall and in that wall are a number of different proteins called antigens or motifs. Unfortunately for us, many of these bacterial antigens are very similar, if not identical, to bits of us. For example, the bacteria implicated in MS have cell wall antigens that look identical to myelin in human nerves. In people with MS, the myelin sheath that coats the nerve cells is attacked by the body's own immune system. *Prevotella copri*, the bacteria implicated in rheumatoid arthritis, has cell wall antigens that look identical to the type 11 collagen contained in human joints. This theory of autoimmune disease pathogenesis is called 'molecular mimicry'. The antigens in bacterial cell wall mimic some of our own bodily tissues and your immune system attacks both the bacteria and you.

However, there is a special type of white blood cell, called a regulatory T cell (Treg). Their job is to keep the immune system under control and deficiencies in Tregs have been associated with autoimmune diseases. The immune cells that make Tregs are located predominantly in the gut. That is a major reason that I believe the gut is the primary site of the development of all autoimmune diseases.

Specific bad gut bugs like segmented filamentous bacteria (SFB) have been shown to change the normal balance of the gut immune system by increasing inflammatory signals that induce attacks on T cells and reduce the anti-inflammatory Treg cells. This increases our ability to fight off intestinal infections. However, this also increases proinflammatory chemicals that may also render us more susceptible to chronic autoimmune inflammation.

| Gut bacteria | Associated autoimmune disease |
|---|---|
| *Streptococcus mitis* | Type 1 diabetes |
| *Klebsiella, Proteus* | Ankylosing spondylitis |
| *Proteus, Prevotella copri, Porphyromonas gingivalis* | Rheumatoid arthritis |
| *Yersinia* | Graves' disease, Hashimoto's thyroiditis |
| *Campylobacter* | Guillain-Barré syndrome |
| *Methanobrevibacter smithii, Chlamydia* | Multiple sclerosis |
| *Novosphingobium* | Primary biliary cirrhosis |
| *E. coli* | Systemic lupus erythematosus, Sjögren's syndrome |

The medical journals accept that, in genetically susceptible people, gut bacteria trigger damage and loss of your immune system's ability to tolerate part of yourself.[41] Excessive contact with bacteria may induce a proinflammatory immune response that, if chronic, can lead to autoimmune disease. Once activated in the gut, T cells recruit antibody-producing immune B cells. B cells transform into autoantibody-producing factories called plasma cells that are responsible for a range of cross-reacting antibodies. You can have your blood tested for a whole panel of recognised autoantibodies. These tests show that many people who are walking around with positive blood tests for one or more of autoantibodies are perfectly well and have no signs of autoimmune disease.

---

[41]  Kostic AD et al, 2014, 'The microbiome in inflammatory bowel disease: current status and the future ahead', *Gastroenterology*, 146(6) pp. 1489-99.

But there's a catch. According to research, the appearance of these autoantibodies in the blood occurs anywhere from four to fourteen years before the onset of autoimmune disease. Once you have an autoantibody being made by your immune system, there is a high chance of developing autoimmune disease in the future. This means that specific bacterial antigens are getting through your gut, triggering a lack of tolerance and mimicking your own tissue. When you are antibody positive, the prediction that you will go on to develop autoimmune disease ranges from 29-100%. Not everyone is going to get sick, but plenty are. The strongest predictor described so far is anticentromere antibody, which has a positive predictive value for the development of SLE of 100% and a time lag from the appearance of the antibody to diagnosis of 11 years.[42]

We should keep in mind that, apart from altered gut bacteria and genetic susceptibility, there must be other factors involved in autoimmune disease development. Genetic susceptibility and gut dysbiosis are both extremely common but autoimmunity is not. Millions of people carry susceptibility genes and have intestinal dysbiosis but only a small fraction of these develop autoimmune diseases. For example, 78% of people with MS have an overgrowth of *Methanobrevibacter smithii* but 31% who are normal also carry it.[43]

Evidence has emerged that implicates a third hit – altered intestinal barrier function or permeability from dysfunction of the tight junctions. While this is still a theory, it is a very attractive one that ticks all boxes in terms of the observed changes associated with autoimmune disease. The tight junctions are sophisticated gatekeeper structures that control the trafficking of molecules across the gut and into our bodies. Lying in wait beneath the surface of the intestine is the enormous gut immune system and nervous system that is constantly sampling what the tight junctions let slip through. They are permanently on the lookout for dangerous bacteria, toxins and poisons. It's the gut barrier working with the gut immune system that controls the delicate balance between what is tolerated and what is attacked whenever a non-self-antigen or molecule is moved through a tight junction.[44]

If you break down that barrier, it allows more antigens or molecules from the gut to flood into the body. In this instance, the gut immune system is suddenly swamped with an abnormally high load of foreign chemicals. The response to this by the gut immune system can be overwhelming, to say the least. They get the

[42] Shoenfeld Y et al, 2008, 'The mosaic of autoimmunity: prediction, autoantibodies, and therapy in autoimmune disease,' *Israel Medical Association Journal*, vol. 10, no. 1, pp. 13, 19.

[43] Ray S et al, 2012, 'Autoimmune disorders: an overview of molecular and cellular basis in today's perspective', *Journal of Clinical & Cellular Immunology*, S10-003.

[44] Fasano A & Shea-Donohue T, 2005, 'Mechanisms of disease: the role of intestinal barrier function in the pathogenesis of gastrointestinal autoimmune diseases', *Nature Clinical Practice Gastroenterology & Hepatology*, vol. 2, no. 9, pp. 416r422.

signal that there are large numbers of foreigners getting through the gut and decide that they must be under attack.[45]

Defective epithelial barrier function, which can be measured as increased intestinal permeability, has been implicated in inflammatory bowel disease (IBD) and can predict relapse during clinical remission.

What else induces leaky gut? As we discussed earlier, it was recently discovered that *Vibrio cholerae*, the bacteria that causes disease cholera, secretes an enterotoxin called zonula occludens toxin (Zot). Zot causes leaky gut by opening up tight junction gaps between gut-lining cells. This finding led to the discovery of zonulin. Zonulin is made by our own gut-lining cells, the enterocytes. It interacts with a specific receptor on the surface of the same enterocytes that make it. When zonulin binds to this receptor it activates an enzyme that opens up the tight junctions, making the gut more leaky.

Zonulin release is stimulated by dysbiotic gut bacteria and by gluten. Zonulin levels are elevated in the tissues and blood of people with autoimmune diseases. A growing number of diseases, including autoimmune diseases, are known to involve alterations in intestinal permeability related to changes in tight junction competency. Zonulin also regulators blood brain barrier permeability.

Medical literature has been publishing work on zonulin for eight years. In 2006, this was published in the journal *Diabetes*:

> Zonulin, a protein that modulates intestinal permeability, is upregulated in several autoimmune diseases and is involved in the pathogenesis of autoimmune diabetes. Zonulin upregulation seems to precede the onset of the disease, providing a possible link between increased intestinal permeability, environmental exposure to non-self antigens, and the development of autoimmunity in the genetically susceptible.[46]

This study implicated the role of zonulin in the development of type 1 diabetes. They took 339 patients with diabetes and compared them to 97 controls and 89 people who had close relatives with diabetes. They found that the diabetics had high levels of zonulin and abnormal intestinal permeability compared to the healthy control subjects. Of the non-diabetic relatives 70% had high zonulin levels and abnormal gut permeability too. The relatives with leaky gut were followed for several years, and 60% of them became diabetic compared with ones who did not have leaky gut.

The study concluded that abnormal intestinal permeability might allow *Streptococcus mites* – bacterial antigens that look identical to the insulin-secreting cells of the pancreas – through the gut barrier, triggering the production of cross-

---

[45]   Caricilli A et al, 2014, 'Intestinal barrier: a gentlemen barrier: a, e Gastroenterology & inflammatory', *World Journal of Gastrointestinal Pathophysiology*, vol. 5, no. 1, pp. 18.32.

[46]   Sapone A et al, 2006, 'Zonulin upregulation is associated with increased gut permeability in subjects with type 1 diabetes and their relatives', *Diabetes*, 55( 5), pp. 1443-1449.

reacting antibodies. In people with genetic susceptibility to diabetes, this is a huge problem. *S. mites* trigger the acquired immune system's T cells to form into attack cells. These guys stimulate B cells, which produce antibodies against *S. mites* that cross-react with antigens on cells of the pancreas, causing inflammation of the insulin-producing cells in the pancreas. If it goes on for long enough, permanent damage to the pancreas occurs and the result is diabetes.

This process has been identified in most autoimmune diseases. Published studies have identified specific bacterial strains that have cell wall motifs that are identical to human tissues that are attacked in autoimmune diseases. We have also identified the specific autoantibodies that have been produced to fight those bacteria, but that cross-react with our own tissues.

There is plenty of support for this theory of autoimmune pathogenesis in the medical literature. Some researches even take it a step further by looking at whether probiotic therapy could change the course of autoimmune disease, which is what this book is all about.[47]

Probiotics may find themselves playing a therapeutic role in the treatment of autoimmune diseases for a couple of reasons. We know that probiotics can help regulate the composition of the intestinal microflora. Specific species of *Lactobacillus* have been shown to stimulate good functioning of gut tight junctions and improve and protect gut barrier function. The actions of gliadin, a protein found in gluten that stimulates zonulin release, opens tight junctions and changes gut permeability, can be blocked in vitro by *Lactobacillus rhamnosus*. Taking this probiotic when you eat gluten could stop any increase in gut permeability. This has yet to be proven in humans. Another probiotic strain, *Lactobacillus plantarum*, has been shown to reduce intestinal permeability. It does this by stimulating the expression of many different genes involved in making the components that form the structure of tight junctions.

The use of probiotics as clinical treatment for autoimmune diseases is yet to be proven effective in humans, but the studies are coming. If this three-hit theory turns out to be right, it will totally change the way we approach the treatment of all autoimmune diseases.

---

[47] Ozdemir O, 2013, 'Any role for probiotics in the therapy or prevention of autoimmune diseases? Up-to-date review', *Journal of Complementary and Integrative Medicine*, vol. 10, no. 1.

# Chapter 25

## Gut bacteria and inflammatory bowel disease

Inflammatory bowel diseases (IBD) like ulcerative colitis and Crohn's disease were once very rare disorders. In Western societies, cases began to rise dramatically in the second half of the 20th century. Recent history has seen the number of cases doubling every decade. IBDs have also expanded into developing countries in the past two decades. As our gut microbiomes become more westernised, it seems our risk of IBD increases.

Let's apply the three-hit hypothesis to ulcerative colitis and Crohn's disease, starting with genetic predisposition. We now have an increased ability to study complete genetic codes. These studies have identified a second type of genetic susceptibility called single nucleotide polymorphisms (SNP). SNPs are very small genetic mutations. So far, more than 160 SNPs have been found that are significantly associated with IBD. They all encode for different alterations in the way our gut immune system distinguishes good from bad bacteria, how trigger-happy the gut lymphocytes are and how permeable the gut lining is.

In Crohn's disease and ulcerative colitis, the recognition and tolerance of our good probiotic gut bacterial community is mediated by special receptors. These are called toll-like receptors and NOD-like receptors. If you carry some of these susceptibility genes, gut bacterial dysbiosis and altered gut permeability can result in the inappropriate activation of these receptors. Once activated, they initiate a cascade of inflammatory signals telling the gut immune system not to tolerate the gut microbiome anymore. The result is a raging immune response to our own gut microbiome with gut inflammation and damage. This is the hallmark of the abnormal intestinal inflammatory response to gut bacteria in Crohn's disease and ulcerative colitis.

The second hit in the theory of autoimmune pathogenesis is exposure to dysbiotic gut bacteria. Studies have confirmed that IBD is caused by changes in the composition of the intestinal microbiota. What the studies have reported in Crohn's disease is an overabundance of Enterobacteriaceae, mostly *E. coli* and *Ruminococcus gnavus* with the loss of *Faecalibacterium prausnitzii*. In particular, *Faecalibacterium prausnitzii* is very important in the setting of Crohn's disease. It is a butyrate-producing bacterium, which means it is a key player in gut lining repair and maintenance and has powerful anti-inflammatory properties. The gut dysbiosis associated with ulcerative colitis is marked by a reduction in biodiversity with low Bacteroidetes and Firmicutes species coupled with overgrowths of *Fusobacterium varium* and *E coli*. Experts now agree that the cause of IBD is the loss of the normal regulation of the gut immune system, which produces an abnormal immune response by the gut against the resident gut flora.[48]

Thirdly, Crohn's disease and ulcerative colitis are now also considered to be permeability disorders. Since the 1980s, studies have implicated abnormal increased permeability in IBD. Patients with IBD show specific abnormalities in tight junction function that is independent of the epithelial damage seen in active colitis. In other words, they have dysfunctional gut permeability that has nothing to do with the ulceration of the gut lining.[49] High intestinal permeability has been shown to predict the risk of relapse in patients with IBD. Patients who are in remission but who still have evidence of leaky gut have an 81% risk of relapse in one year compared to 17% of those with normal permeability.[50]

Despite all this evidence, the current medical approach to IBD treatment continues to focus entirely on immunosuppressant drugs. Gut dysbiosis and permeability are still ignored and treatment aimed at restoring the health of the intestinal microbiome is non-existent.

We know there are several strains of probiotic bacteria than can modulate the gut immune system by increasing Tregs and reducing the cytokine that drives much of the inflammation in IBD. These include *Lactobacillus rhamnosus GG*, *Bifidobacterium lactis*, *Saccharomyces boulardii* and the probiotic blend called VSL#3. Studies of probiotics used to treat IBD have been promising in theory but disappointing in practice, with only modest improvements that are short-lived.[51]

However, there is one shining light on the horizon and that is faecal transplant. The process of taking a load of gut microbes from a healthy person's poo and squirting it up the bowel of a person with IBD is showing great promise. This treatment is designed to change the composition of the gut microbiome and preliminary studies are showing great promise.

The largest and most exciting study was performed in Sydney. Forty-one adults with moderately severe ulcerative colitis that was resistant to standard drug treatment were given five faecal microbiota transplants (FMT) every week for eight weeks. The FMTs were multi-donor transplants, meaning that each transplant was made by mixing stool taken from between three and seven different donors who were unrelated to the recipient. Eight weeks after FMT treatment, 41% of the patients were in complete clinical remission and off all steroid drugs, compared with 20% of those receiving placebos. This result was big news in the

[48]  Strober W et al, 2007, 'The fundamental basis of inflammatory bowel disease', *Journal of Clinical Investigation*, vol. 117, no. 3, pp. 514-521.

[49]  Arnott ID et al, 2000, 'Abnormal intestinal permeability predicts relapse in inactive Crohn disease', *Scandinavian Journal of Gastroenterology*, vol. 35, issue 11; pp. 1163-1169.

[50]  Wyatt J et al, 1993, 'Intestinal permeability and the prediction of relapse in Crohn's disease', *The Lancet*, vol. 341, no. 8858, pp. 1437, 1439.

[51]  Scaldaferri F et al, 2013, 'Gut microbial flora, prebiotics, and probiotics in ibd: their current usage and utility', *BioMed Research International*, vol. 2013, article ID 435268.

gastro world and the study was selected for presentation at the European Crohn's and Colitis Organisation 2016 Congress in Amsterdam.[52]

An exciting pilot study of FMT in Crohn's disease was published in 2015. The researchers looked at 30 patients who had failed to respond to any drug therapy. They gave them all an FMT into the small intestine. Four weeks later, 76.7% of these Crohn's disease patients were in clinical remission and free from symptoms. FMT allowed them to gain weight and improved their cholesterol as well.[53]

One of my patients, Steven, whom I treated with faecal transplant therapy for resistant ulcerative colitis in the context of his Parkinson's disease, has written about the treatment in his inspirational book *Finding Hope: When Facing Serious Disease*.

> The first thing I noticed was my colon felt settled, more settled than it had felt in years. In the five years since I had developed ulcerative colitis, a background irritability threatening and/or developing into a bowel motion was with me most of the time. Now it was gone. In the initial weeks following FMT my bowel felt foreign to me. Rather than colitis, with its characteristic loose stools, the first two months were characterised by constipation. The key to managing this was to increase my fibre and water intake. Blissfully, I had none of the mouth ulcers that had plagued me whenever colitis threatened. To our delight my general stamina was also increasing, allowing me to get out and about more without the anxiety of having to rush to the nearest loo. Two weeks before my recommended three-monthly top-up enema, I did notice an increased bowel irritability which settled following the additional FMT.

[52] Paramothy S et al. Multi-donor intensive faecal microbiota transplantation for active ulcerative colitis: a randomised placebo-controlled trial. The Lancet 2017; 389no 10075: 1218-1228.

[53] Cui B et al, 2015, 'Fecal microbiota transplantation through mid-gut for refractory Crohn's disease: safety, feasibility, and efficacy trial results', *Journal of Gastroenterology and Hepatology*, vol. 30, no. 1, pp. 51en8.

# Chapter 26

# Gut bacteria and systemic lupus erythematosus

Systemic lupus erythematosus (SLE) – also known as lupus – is another common autoimmune disease that is on the rise. Its incidence has tripled in the last 50 years. SLE makes life hell for sufferers because it doesn't just attack joints. It also spreads to the skin, kidneys, heart, lung, and brain. The symptoms of SLE include pain or swelling in the joints, muscle aches, heartburn, acid reflux, fevers, red facial rashes, chest pains, hair loss, pale or purple fingers or toes, sensitivity to the sun, swelling in legs or around eyes, mouth ulcers, swollen glands and fatigue.

SLE affects more than two million Americans and it discriminates by sex. Nine out of 10 cases of SLE occur in women aged 15 to 45, but men start to catch up once they are over 50 years of age. As with all autoimmune diseases, doctors take the line that the cause is unknown, but we all agree that more and more evidence is pointing towards as a potential factor being changes in the microbes of the gut triggering dysregulation of the immune system.

Several studies in animal models of SLE have shown dysbiosis of the normal healthy gut microbiome. They have consistently found that, just prior to disease onset, lactic acid bacteria *Lactobacillus* are depleted while Clostridial Lachnospiraceae species are over-represented.

In people with SLE, a recent cross-sectional study has found that they have lower-than-accepted normal ratios of Firmicutes to Bacteroidetes and Firmicutes to Proteobacteria than healthy people. Probiotics from the Firmicutes phylum make butyrate, which actively promotes the formation of Tregs, the immune-calming white blood cells that actively suppress inflammation.[54]

Certain bacteria, such as *E. coli*, produce a cell wall protein called Ro-60 which triggers attack from the gut immune system. In SLE, one of the main antigens in human tissue that SLE autoantibodies attack is so similar to the bacterial Ro-60 cell wall protein that our immune system can't tell the difference. It will attack any human tissues bearing the biosimilar A/Ro-60 antigen.[55]

Two specific gut bacterial cell wall toxins – lipoteichoic acid and lipopolysaccharide – have been reported to contribute to the initiation and maintenance of SLE. Once in the bloodstream, these bacterial toxins drive

[54] Arpaia N et al, 2013, 'Metabolites produced by commensal bacteria promote peripheral regulatory T-cell generation', *Nature* , vol. 504, no. 7480, pp. 451-455; Smith PM et al, 2013, 'The microbial metabolites, short-chain fatty acids, regulate colonic Treg cell homeostasis', *Science*, vol. 341, no. 6145, pp. 569-573.

[55] Poole BD et al, 2006, 'Epstein-Barr virus and molecular mimicry in systemic lupus erythematosus', *Autoimmunity*, vol. 39, no. 1, pp. 63 70; Szymula A et al, 2014, 'T cell epitope mimicry between Sjögren's syndrome Antigen A (SSA)/Ro60 and oral, gut, skin and vaginal bacteria', *Clinical Immunology*, vol. 152, pp. 1-9.

receptors on the innate immune cells in the gut absolutely crazy. These receptors recognise invading microorganisms and their toxins, which triggers the acquired immune system to go to war. If any of these bits of bacteria get past your gut lining, they mimic parts of your own tissues. Then you accidently become the target of your own immune system too and SLE is the end result.

In people, external factors such as antibiotics and diet modulate the gut microbiota with a potential impact in SLE. Antibiotics are known to trigger SLE flares in patients. In fact, African-Americans, who are more likely to develop SLE, have used antibiotics much more frequently than other people in Western societies. One suggested mechanism is that antibiotics lead to the decrease of bacterial metabolites that calm down the immunes system and reduce autoimmune attack.[56]

Dietary components can also influence SLE by changing the composition and function of gut microbiota. For example, vitamin D, vitamin A, and omega-3 polyunsaturated fatty acids have been found to modulate SLE onset or flares.[57]

Why is SLE mostly a female disorder? The female hormone oestrogen has been shown to aggravate many autoimmune diseases. We know that the gut microbiomes in male and female rats and humans are significantly different. Male hormones like testosterone have been shown to affect the microbiome. Recent research suggests that the male-type microbiome and male hormones protect male mice from autoimmune disease. When you give SLE-prone female mice a faecal transplant from a healthy male donor it protects them from the disease. Dr Michele Kosiewicz from the University of Louisville believes that the male-type microbiome contains specific probiotic bacteria that make metabolic by-products that modulate gut Tregs.

It turns out that Toll-like receptors, the supercharged stimulators of the immune response, are more sensitive to oestrogen than testosterone. Females with SLE are loaded with far more activated white blood cells that are covered in Toll-like receptors than anybody else.[58]

Finally, a nasty little protein called curli, which dysbiotic bacteria make as part of the biofilm they use to protect themselves, has been shown to trigger autoimmune disease and specifically SLE. Certain *E. coli* and *Salmonella* species make curli. Researchers dropped dendrocytes from the gut into the biofilm made by *Salmonella*. The gut dendrocytes were able to drive their tentacles into the biofilm to grab and start destroying the *Salmonella*, just like they do when *Salmonella* infects the gut. The surprise was that the curli protein in the biofilm was also engulfed by the dendrocytes. This happens because curli latches firmly

---

[56] Rojo D et al, 2015, 'Ranking the impact of human health disorders on gut metabolism: systemic lupus erythematosus and obesity as study cases', *Scientific Reports (Nature)*, vol. 5, 8310.

[57] Mu Q, 2015, 'SLE: Another Autoimmune Disorder influenced by Microbes and Diet?', *Frontiers in Immunology*, vol. 6, article 608.

[58] Jiang W et al, 2014, 'Sex differences in monocyte activation in systemic lupus erythematosus (SLE)', *PLoS ONE*, vol. 9, no. 12, e114589.

onto exposed DNA from the dying *Salmonella*. The dendrocytes then present bits of *Salmonella* together with DNA-curli protein to the T cells of the gut acquired immune system. The curli protein, when combined with *Salmonella* DNA, induced a massive immune over-reaction compared to just the bits of *Salmonella* alone.

The scientists then injected the curli-DNA composite into a strain of mice that is prone to developing SLE. The mice began producing autoantibodies within just two weeks, compared to four or five months for the control mice.

This result indicates that, in SLE-prone mice, exposure to gut bacterial biofilm components can trigger disease. The researchers also showed that even normal mice made autoantibodies in response to curli-DNA complexes, but at much lower levels and much more slowly.

Curli's role in eliciting autoimmunity was confirmed in the next set of experiments, which involved infecting mice with curli-producing bacteria. The researchers infected mice with bacteria that make curli – either *E. coli*, which normally inhabits the gut, or *Salmonella* – and compared the mice's response to that of mice infected with bacteria that lack curli. They found that the curli-producing bacteria led to higher levels of autoantibodies than bacteria that lacked the protein.

Together, these results show that curli, which is made by several types of bacteria that inhabit or infect the gastrointestinal tract, can promote signs of SLE in both SLE-prone and normal mice.[59]

To directly examine the potential effects of sex and gut microbiota on SLE, one approach would be to correct the imbalanced microbial composition associated with SLE with faecal transplantation from male donors and see if this alleviates the disease. This is yet to be reported for SLE patients and remains an area that researchers need to explore actively.

---

[59] Gallo PM et al, 2015, 'Amyloid-DNA composites of bacterial biofilms induce autoimmunity', *Immunity*, vol. 42, no. 6, pp. 171-184.

# Chapter 27

## Gut bacteria and allergies

When I was a younger doctor, still a neophyte when it came to the importance of the gut microbiome, my wife and I decided to have kids. Before long we were the proud parents of a bald, blue-eyed angelic baby boy. We called him Charlie.

Charlie was born by elective caesarean section. My wife, given her past medical history of almost losing her sight when the vision receptors on the back wall of her left eyeball started peeling off like dry paint in the sun for no apparent reason, decided not to go through labour. Spontaneous retinal detachment, if not treated promptly, can lead quickly to blindness. While there is no accepted protocol on what should or shouldn't be done in terms of childbirth after retinal detachment, our obstetrician agreed to an elective caesarean for fear of it happening due to the high abdominal pressures generated in labour. This meant that our newborn son received his first bacterial microbiome from the skin and oral cavities of his parents and everybody else that touched him, rather than from the birth canal.

As luck would have it, my wife was unable to breastfeed so baby Charlie was a formula-fed infant until he started solids at six months of age. Despite this he was a robust toddler until he was three, when we let him eat a piece of chocolate brownie to celebrate his little sister's second birthday. With the brownie still half in his mouth, Charlie's lips began to swell and his cheeks turned a bright shade of scarlet.

I rinsed all traces of the brownie out of his mouth and looked him over. He seemed to be breathing and comfortable. 'It'll be fine,' I reassured my already panic-stricken wife and turned back to the table to take a closer look at the brownie. It turned out there were walnuts in it.

'No, it won't!' my wife blurted back at me, right as Charlie started complaining about his throat closing over.

You can imagine what happened next. After being rushed to hospital, Charlie was given a cocktail of antihistamines and steroids and we were given an appointment to see an allergist. Testing confirmed that Charlie had a severe allergy to tree nuts, which included cashews, walnuts, pistachios, pecans, Brazil nuts and macadamias. He was also allergic to peanuts. The only nuts he didn't react to were hazelnuts and almonds.

Having a child diagnosed with a severe nut allergy is a nightmare. We lived in a perpetual state of abject fear that something as innocent as a peanut might kill our son, and Charlie developed anxiety and fear of food. Our healthy son became a 'special person'. Both my wife and I had to carry antihistamines and an EpiPen of injectable adrenalin on us at all times. Everywhere that Charlie went, whether it was school, parties, camps or sports, he carried a medi-alert to warn everyone who encountered him of his potentially life-threatening nut allergy. We were required to send him with a medi-pack bristling with antihistamines, steroids, emergency telephone numbers and EpiPens in case he ate a nut and started going into anaphylactic shock.

At least we were not alone, the allergist reassured us. A recent Australian study found 10% of 12-month-old babies and 3% of infants have a peanut allergy. Peanut allergies have increased by 350% in the past two decades. It is the most common cause of death due to food allergy.

The incidence of lethal food allergies in Australian kids is skyrocketing. Nowadays, one in 20 children has a food allergy and one in 100 has a severe nut allergy. My friend and paediatric gastroenterologist, Dr Katie Allen, summarised this situation beautifully:

> The 'allergy epidemic' is a major public health issue predominantly facing Western countries, including Australia. There has been a rapid increase over the past 30 years in the prevalence of allergic conditions such as asthma, eczema and food allergy, and the causes remain unknown. Food allergy prevalence in particular has increased dramatically over the past decade. Most concerning is that food allergy is a problem that affects mainly children.[60]

Around 85% of children with an early allergy to foods, including eggs, cow's milk, wheat and soy, will develop tolerance to these foods by the time they are five.[61] But research has shown that allergies to peanuts and tree nuts are typically life-long. Only 20% of children with a peanut allergy and 9% of children with a tree nut allergy outgrew them by the time they reached school.[62]

To explain, a food allergy occurs when your gastrointestinal immune system triggers an inappropriate allergic reaction when you eat a specific food. Essentially, the gut immune system mistakenly treats this food as if it's a toxin or an infection rather than a food, and reacts by making antibodies to fight it off. The symptoms develop because of all the chemicals like histamine that are unleashed upon the hapless food particle. There have been reports of allergic reactions to just about any food. How very reassuring.

'What's the cure?' I asked.

'There is no cure.'

I told our son's allergist that I had read that 5% of children grow out of their nut allergy but his grim-faced response was, 'Kids with severe nut allergies don't

[60] Sicherer SH, 2011, 'Epidemiology of food allergy', *Journal of Allergy and Clinical Immunology*, vol. 127, no. 3, pp. 594 and C

[61] Wood RA, 2003, 'The natural history of food allergy', *Pediatrics*, vol. 111, no. 6, part 3, pp. 163 part 3,

[62] Ho MH et al, 2008, 'Early clinical predictors of remission of peanut allergy in children', *Journal of Allergy and Clinical Immunology*, vol. 121, pp. 731 , by Fleischer DM et al, 2005, 'The natural history of tree nut allergy', *Journal of Allergy and Clinical Immunology*, vol. 116, pp. 108711093.

grow out of them. He'll have it for life.' Charlie was booked in for allergy testing every three years.

Faced with this bleak scenario, I turned to the gut microbiome. I was well aware of the 'hygiene hypothesis' that postulated that clean environments together with the overuse of disinfectants and antibiotics results in kids developing unhealthy and relatively weaker biodiversity in their gut microbiomes than ever before. This seems to correlate well with the explosion of childhood allergies. Probiotics seem like a safe way of boosting the gut microflora, and they just might reduce the incidence of allergy.

Several animal studies have demonstrated that treating animals with probiotics like *Lactobacillus johnsonii* and *Bacteroides fragilis*, together with the short-chain fatty acid propionate, confers significant protection against the development of allergic airway conditions.[63]

When Charlie was 10 years old, his skin prick tests were all still strongly positive. I decided to have a serious go at changing his gut microbiome. For the next year and a half, his diet included big reductions in dairy, wheat and sugar, more prebiotic foods like onion, garlic, beetroot, spinach, kale and broccoli, and some fermented foods such as yoghurts with live cultures. I also supplemented him with a daily dose of specific probiotic strains that have been implicated in studies as being able to modify allergies. Finally, I added a blend of bovine colostrum mixed with Immunoglobulin A, Immunoglobulin G, lactoferrin, larch, selenium, iodine and zinc to boost his gut mucosal barrier. It was not an easy task. But I soon discovered that he would guzzle down a cup full of fresh broccoli, kale and baby spinach leaves if I tossed them in a blender filled with almond milk, frozen blueberries, frozen raspberries, a teaspoon of organic cocoa powder, bovine colostrum and ice. He loved this smoothie and gulped down his probiotic capsules easily with it.

Life went on as usual until, about a year later, my wife rang my office, her agitation palpable. 'It's Charlie,' she said. I immediately thought he'd eaten a nut and died.

'Is he in hospital? Is he alive?'

'He's fine. The allergy nurse did his skin prick test today and they all came up negative!'

I didn't believe it. 'What did the allergist say?'

'She said it must be a mistake, and she made the nurse do it again with a fresh batch of nut sera and double the dose.'

This would effectively be three times the recommended safe dose for skin prick testing and should have set him off like a fire cracker.

'And?'

'Nothing happened again!'

---

[63]  Panzer AR & Lynch SV, 2015, 'Influence and effect of the human microbiome in allergy and asthma', *Current Opinion in Rheumatology*, vol. 27, no. 4, pp. 373 R80.

I could hardly believe what I was hearing.

'What did the allergist say that time?'

'She still doesn't believe it, so she's taken a blood test to check it out.'

Two days later my wife was back at the allergists for the results. Amazingly, the blood tests came back negative. The allergist still couldn't believe it but, faced with the irrefutable test results, she decided to book Charlie into hospital for nut challenges.

Over the next few weeks, Charlie fronted up to hospital where, surrounded by doctors, nurses, intravenous drugs, resuscitation trolleys and oxygen masks, he munched his way through bag after bag of every different kind of nut in the food chain. He did all of this without any sort of reaction at all. At his final appointment with the allergist, the doctor told Charlie he was no longer allergic to nuts. She told my wife that she could safely throw away the antihistamines and the EpiPen. In her excitement, my wife told the allergist that I had put Charlie on a regime of probiotics, prebiotics and bovine colostrum to help retrain his immune system and reduce his gut permeability. The allergist just smiled.

'That had nothing to do with it.'

My wife cocked her head, raised an eyebrow and gave the doctor one of her 'You're full of shit' glares that she frequently throws my way when she thinks I'm completely in the wrong.

'You're telling me that you – a doctor and allergy physician – are putting this cure down to a "miracle" rather than entertain the slightest possibility that the therapeutic manipulation of the gut microbiome might have had anything to do with it?'

The allergist nodded. 'That's exactly what I'm saying.'

My wife then asked the doctor if she had read Associate Professor Mimi Tang's research paper on probiotic treatment of nut allergies. The allergist shrugged.

'Well, maybe you should,' said my wife as she marched Charlie out of the allergist's office for the last time.

Whether it was a 'miracle', whether it was my gut microbiome treatment or whether he just grew out of it, we will never know. But given what we know about how gut bacteria train the gut immune system about what is safe to eat and what is not, the epidemic of childhood food allergies urgently needs to be thought about and researched in terms of the role of the gut microbiome. Throwing away that EpiPen was one of the happiest days of my life. If this book can help start others on the journey to do the same, I will be ecstatic.

In 2015, Professor Tang's group from the Murdoch Children's Research Institute in Melbourne theorised that a particular strain of probiotics might have a role in retraining the gut immune system in kids with life-threatening peanut allergies. They gave 60 peanut-allergic kids aged less than 10 either a probiotic plus peanut protein or a placebo.

Tang was staggered by the results. Two to five weeks after treatment had finished, over 80% of children who received the probiotics and peanut protein were no longer allergic to peanuts, compared with only 7.1% who received a placebo.

'This is 20 times higher than the natural rate of resolution for peanut allergy,' Tang said in an interview. No wonder she was shocked.

The particular strain of probiotic Tang used in the study was exactly the same probiotic strain that I had been giving my son for the previous two years: *Lactobacillus rhamnosus*.

'We have modified the allergic response to peanuts by changing the make-up of gut bacteria,' Tang said. Her paper is worth a read.[64]

There is lots of evidence to suggest that exposure to antibiotics as an infant is involved in the development of what doctors call 'atopy'. Atopy is a collective medical term for allergic disorders like asthma, eczema, hay fever and food allergies. It is thought that the antibiotics cause a deleterious change in the composition of infant gut microbiota and that this is the major trigger for the loss of tolerance and the abnormal allergic immune response.

Research is now implicating altered gut bacteria in asthma and allergies, specifically increases in coliforms and *Staphylococcus* together with decreased *Lactobacillus* and *Bifidobacterium*, and continuing to show benefit of specific *Lactobacillus* probiotic strains in switching off asthma and food allergies.[65]

More recently, the Swansea Baby Trial demonstrated that probiotics significantly reduced the chance of babies developing allergies and eczema. This was the 'full monty' in terms of hard-core medical research. It was a randomised, double-blind, placebo-controlled study of 454 mother-baby pairs who were given a placebo or a high-dose multi-strain probiotic blend of 10 billion organisms daily. The pregnant women took the probiotic from 36 weeks of gestation until delivery. The newborns were given the probiotic from birth until six months of age. At two years of age, those babies whose mothers and themselves took the probiotics had a 44% reduction in common allergies and a 57% reduction in atopic eczema. This was irrefutable proof that the composition of gut bacteria early in life significantly influences allergy. Exposure to sufficient levels of the right types of gut bacteria appears to be critical in steering the immune system away from becoming 'allergic'.[66]

Many experts also believe that leaky gut plays a role in the development of food allergies. Physicians are just now beginning to recognise the importance of the gastrointestinal tract and intestinal permeability in the development of allergic

[64] Tang ML et al, 2015, 'Administration of a probiotic with peanut oral immunotherapy: a randomized trial', *Journal of Allergy and Clinical Immunology*, vol. 135, no. 3, pp. 737.744.

[65] Kang YB et al, 2016, 'Gut microbiota and allergy/asthma: from pathogenesis to new therapeutic strategies', *Allergologia et Immunopathologia*, vol. 45, no. 3, pp. 305tholo

[66] The Swansea Baby Trial, http://lab4probiotics.co.uk/the-swansea-baby-trial/index.html, viewed 22 June 2017.

or autoimmune diseases. Maybe treating the abnormal gut bacteria may turn out to be the final solution in reversing these abnormal states of immune activation. This story from one of my patients illustrates just that.

Mrs TS - Let me begin with my symptoms: I had multiple allergies including itchy eczema from birth. I developed asthma that emerged in puberty, along with anxiety and depression. Then, in my late teens, the onset of chronic fatigue syndrome took hold.

I was one of those children; pale skin, circles under my eyes, eczema on my mouth, inner elbows, scalp and back of the knees. Emotionally, I was a reactive child, and school wasn't easy. Then puberty hit, and my "allergies" got worse; now cognitive (brain fog) and fatigue issues were a big problem. High school was also difficult. I never really thrived; my final year's marks, however, were good enough to get me into uni.

I won't drag out all the details, save to say by the time I was 24, I'd dropped out of uni and was in a desperate state. Emotionally I was quite dysfunctional, eczema blanketed my entire body, particularly my face, and I also struggled with night sweats, constant fatigue and body aches.

My then-boyfriend found a book detailing the symptoms of multiple allergic disorder, and from that, we found an allergy specialist: Dr Colin Little. He admitted me into hospital for 10 weeks, where I was treated in a specialised allergy clinic in which all the environmental variables were filtered and regulated; think of girl in a bubble. After being in a trigger-free environment and fasting for five days, I was a different person; my eczema was disappearing, and I looked and felt much better.

During those 10 weeks, Dr Little established that I was allergic to nearly everything, but with a particularly low tolerance to car exhaust emissions, bleach, perfumes, moulds, dust mites and various grasses.

With the help of my extremely supportive family, we modified the house somewhat and also purchased portable HEPA filters for my bedroom and office. Nearly everything about my diet and the way I lived needed changing.

After implementing all the changes we could reasonably implement – as I wasn't going to live in a bubble all my life, I improved enough to start working for my dad; he gave me the time I needed to sleep and recover, on average I could work 20-40 hrs per week. Keep in mind, however, I lived and worked most of the time at my parents' home, and attended to little or no domestic work (thank you, Mum). In real terms, I had 20-40 hours of energy per week to meet my life's obligations. Worse than that, the energy levels I describe were by no means constant; any trigger could leave me fairly useless for a couple of days. This cycle lasted for approximately 16 years.

I was now 42, and during a low point in October 2014, I watched a BBC medical program that included a segment on FMT. I made an appointment to see Dr Froomes that week. He did some tests and advised that I had leaky gut and potential thyroid issues. He suggested FMT, noting that he had some anecdotal evidence of its success, but could promise nothing. Owing to cost concerns and also the stupid amount of money that I'd spent on health treatments that, in the past, hadn't worked, I didn't immediately commence the treatment. Nonetheless, the articles on FMT continued to mount, and the buzz kept getting more interesting...

By late August 2017, I knew I had to try it. I talked it over with my GP and was booked in for late October 2017, receiving one FMT infusion via colonoscopy and 10 subsequent infusions via a self-administered enema, all occurring within a two-and-a-half-week period. On day three of my first treatment I felt different – calmer, my thoughts were clearer, and, weirdly, my skin felt very soft and smooth. Something was happening, but realistically it was too soon to say. By day five I was sick, very sick. I had a temperature, a terrible sinus infection, body aches – I was bedridden for five to seven days. By day 20, I was feeling much better and could work again and was getting excited about the results. When I say excited, I mean very excited.

It is three months since my initial treatment, and I have supplementary FMT infusions twice a month. Happily, I've tolerated the allergy season better than any previous year. I am no longer anxious or depressed and can work, consistently, full time and complete my domestic chores. Importantly, I still take an antidepressant, but before my FMT treatment, anxiety and low mood were weak points, even on meditation.

Any person suffering CFS with multiple allergy symptoms should consider this treatment, and I say this with a smile; please balance your expectations, FMT isn't a miracle cure. Currently, I think I am at 75-85% of my full capacity, so I'm still recovering, and as suggested by Dr Froomes, I maintain a reasonably strict diet. I've been ill for most of my life, and something of that magnitude doesn't change overnight, but, now I consider it a matter of time rather than never. I will recover and find full health or something close enough to it.

Thank you to Dr Froomes for this innovative treatment, you've been a kind and supportive practitioner.

Finally, a big thank you to all the other people, including Dr Colin Little, my partner, my brother, and my remarkable parents, who have helped me throughout my very long journey. Honestly, I wouldn't be here without you.

With much love and, now, hope!


Another tool in the fight against allergy may be colostrum – a nursing mother's first milk. It is perfect for a newborn animal or human that has minimal gut defences because it is bursting with protective antibodies. By drinking colostrum the newborn receives immune defences and other components that build probiotic bacteria and reduce the intestinal permeability. All of this protects against allergens and pathogens and helps the infant immune system tolerate its environment and not become allergic to it.

Research shows that bovine colostrum may benefit humans with allergies. Bovine colostrum, like human colostrum, contains components that are important in the process of developing a normal immune response. Bovine colostrum passively transfers components that delay and reduce hypersensitivity. According to recent research, proline-rich polypeptide (PRP) from colostrum can work as a regulatory substance of the thymus gland. It has been shown to eliminate or improve the symptoms of allergies, as well as other autoimmune diseases such as MS, rheumatoid arthritis and SLE.

Hopefully, research will soon lead to the end of allergies through appropriate correction of the specific imbalances of the gut microbiome that trigger the immune system into inappropriate action. But there is much you can safely do right now to regrow your own healthy gut microbiome.

# Chapter 28

## Gut bacteria, skin and hair

Mike is a retired fire services officer, aged 63. He came to me complaining of chronic eczema and decades of bloating, wind and 'very unpredictable, crappy bowels'. He basically spent his days swinging between diarrhoea and cramping or constipation and bloating, never knowing what was coming his way from one day to the next.

When I asked Mike about his diet, he confessed that white bread made his bloating and constipation worse and a single sandwich made from two slices of white bread would cause his eczema to break out like crazy the next day. This happened so regularly that his doctor prescribed him a steroid cream to use if he found himself in a situation where he was unable to avoid eating white bread. All his tests for coeliac disease came back negative.

I put Mike on a gut reload program, which included a gluten-free microbiome-boosting diet with prebiotic and probiotic supplementation. Within four weeks his gut symptoms had abated and his rashes had cleared. After eight weeks, his reaction to bread had completely disappeared. I still cautioned him to avoid bread, as chronic exposure leads to altered permeability, which could trigger his skin reactions again.

A group of Spanish dermatologists have demonstrated higher levels of a specific gut bacterial-derived toxin called lipopolysaccharide (LPS) in the blood of patients with psoriasis who also have metabolic syndrome (high blood sugar, excess body fat, elevated blood pressure and cholesterol). LPS is a sugar that is part of the cell membrane of a large number of bacteria that live within the gut. Finding elevated LPS levels in the bloodstream is an indication of two things. First, it means that the gut has become permeable or leaky, which has allowed LPS to get into the bloodstream. Second, it means that the process of inflammation has been enhanced. LPS acts as a powerful switch, turning on the inflammatory cascade. Even when the skin condition improved using phototherapy (a treatment targeted at the skin), the levels of LPS did not change. The phototherapy was treating the smoke but ignoring the fire.[67]

Eczema causes patches of itchy, red, cracked and dry skin. It's basically chronic inflammation of the superficial layers of the skin. It's also referred to as atopic dermatitis, or atopic eczema. A recent study of more than 300,000 children and teenagers in 51 different countries found that they were more likely to

---

[67] Romaní J et al, 2012, 'Lipopolysaccharide-binding protein is increased in patients with psoriasis with metabolic syndrome, and correlates with C-reactive protein,' *Clinical and Experimental Dermatology*, vol. 38, no. 1, pp. 81-84.

develop asthma, hay fever and eczema if they ate fast food three or more times a week over a 12-month period.[68]

Another study looked at children with eczema and those without eczema when they were six and eighteen months old and compared their gut microbiota. Results showed that all the infants had the same types of bacteria at six months. However, by 18 months, the toddlers with eczema had more of a type of bacteria known as *Clostridium* clusters IV and XIVa, which are usually linked to adults. The kids who were not affected by eczema had higher quantities of the probiotic Bacteroidetes.

The researchers concluded:

*The composition of bacteria in a child's gut depends on its environment and the food it eats. You would expect that as a child's diet changes, so will the bacteria present. The number of bifidobacteria naturally falls with age and in total we found 21 groups of bacteria, which changed in this time period. However, it is the early change towards adult-type bacteria which seems to be a risk factor for eczema.*

In my practice, almost everyone who has FMT for bowel problems reports that their skin clears up. They don't complain about skin problems at their consultations, but it has become apparent that skin problems are quite common in many gut illnesses. When I began to ask my patients about their skin, I was surprised to find out that they all suffered from skin complaints that included eczema, dry flaky skin, intermittent rashes, acne, rosacea, redness and itching. This is an area that deserves close attention and more research.

As bizarre as it seems, your resident bowel bugs seem to have something to do with regrowing your hair. At least if your hair loss is due to the autoimmune disease called Alopecia Areata. In this condition, your own immune system attacks and destroys your hair follicles, leaving sufferers not only bald but also at risk of losing not just the hair on their head but all body hair.

A case report has been published describing two people with Alopecia Areata both of whom had also contracted the nasty bowel infection called *Clostridium difficile*. Their physician treated them with gut microbiome restoration therapy by faecal transplant.[69]

FMT, as expected, successfully eradicated the bowel infections but surprisingly both patients found that their hair started to grow back. One of them, who had been completely hairless for over 10 years, grew hair on his face, arms and scalp

---

[68]  Ellwood P et al, 2013, 'Do fast foods cause asthma, rhinoconjunctivitis and eczema? Global findings from the International Study of Asthma and Allergies in Childhood (ISAAC) Phase Three', *Thorax*, vol. 68, pp. 351-360.

[69]  Rebello D et al. Hair Growth in Two Alopecia Patients after Fecal Microbiota Transplant. ACG Case Reports Journal; 2017; 4e:107.

to about 50% of his pre-alopecia hair levels. The evidence linking an unhealthy gut microbiome and autoimmune disease continues to grow more compelling.

# Chapter 29

## Gut bacteria and mood

When Karen, a tired, anxious and single 27-year-old office worker, walked into my consulting rooms complaining of bloating, cramping and bouts of constipation alternating with diarrhoea that were ruining her life, I simply nodded in agreement.

'That's not the usual response I get from doctors,' she remarked. 'And don't try to tell me it's in my head either.'

'No, it's in your gut,' I replied. 'And I'm going to prove it to you with a stool test and then we are going to fix it.'

She cried tears of joy. She readily agreed to change her diet and undergo a course of FMTs to turn her dysbiotic microbiome into a probiotic one. She wanted a female donor and I was happy to oblige.

She visited my office again four weeks after completing her FMT treatments. She sat down in the chair opposite my desk and smiled.

'Doc, what have you done to me?'

'Hopefully, fixed your irritable bowel,' I answered.

'Oh, my bowels are fine now,' she said. 'But I've had a complete personality transplant! Before the transplant, I was a bit of a recluse. I never went out to work functions, never had drinks after work with the girls and never went on dates with guys. In the space of four weeks I've turned into a party girl! It's so out of character for me. I'm out at every social function I can find. I go for drinks after work all the time and I'm the life of the party. I love it. My friends can't believe I'm the same girl.'

That was a new one on me. But the change was clearly visible and very real for her. I looked up her donor. She was unrelated, 23 years old and also an office worker. She was into health, described herself as a very bubbly and outgoing person who had a lot of friends and was very social.

The idea that swarms of bacteria living in the gut can alter personality and mood has stunned the medical profession. Human studies are being published proving that the gut microbiome has powerful effects on the brain and mood. So impressive is this link that gut bacteria are now being referred to as 'psychobiotics' instead of probiotics.

The brain and the gut enteric nervous system are extraordinarily well connected. While many people believe their brain is the organ in charge of their body, the gut sends far more information to the brain than the brain sends to the gut.

To put this into more concrete terms, you've probably experienced the unsettling sensation of butterflies in your stomach when you're nervous, or felt like you had a knot in your stomach when you are very angry or stressed. You may also have noticed that an upset tummy brings on anxiety and low mood. Medical science has proven that an imbalance in your gut microbes can directly impact your mental health, leading to issues like anxiety, depression and altered behaviour.

Probiotics have been found to improve mood. To date, most of the research has been conducted on mice. Feeding mice *Lactobacillus rhamnosus* made them less stressed and reduced depressive behaviours when they were forced to swim after being dropped in water. *Lactobacillus reuteri* promoted the release of oxytocin in mice – our body's 'love potion' hormone – and was shown to give the animals a 'glow of health'.[70]

One fascinating study demonstrated that baby mice with symptoms that resemble autism in humans have had those symptoms reversed after being given *Bacteroides fragilis*, suggesting (at least in this mouse model) that the symptoms of autism may be reversible with probiotic therapy.[71]

There have been studies on people too. Drinking a probiotic mixture containing *Lactobacillus helveticus* and *Bifidobacterium longum* for 30 days has beneficial effects on anxiety and depressive measures, as well as reduced levels of the stress hormone cortisol.[72]

Healthy women who drank a fermented milk product containing four particular species of bacteria (*Bifidobacterium animalis*, *Streptococcus thermophilus*, *Lactobacillus bulgaricus* and *Lactococcus lactis*) for four weeks were shown to have alterations in brain regions that control emotion and pain sensation.[73]

A study of chronic fatigue syndrome (CFS) patients found that a two-month course of probiotics led to a significant decrease in their symptoms of depression and anxiety. The researchers administered 39 CFS patients either three doses of *Lactobacillus casei Shirota* or a placebo every day for two months. They found that 73% of subjects taking the probiotic experienced an increase in levels of *Lactobacillus* and *Bifidobacterium* in the gut, which corresponded with a significant decrease in anxiety symptoms. The positive calming effect of the probiotics was mediated by increasing the levels of the feel-good chemical tryptophan. They also reported big improvements in gut pain and bloating. In the placebo group, only 37.5% showed an increase in *Bifidobacterium*, while only

---

[70] Poutahidis T et al, 2013. 'Microbial symbionts accelerate wound healing via the neuropeptide hormone oxytocin', *PLoS ONE*, vol. 8, no. 10, e78898.

[71] Hanely S et al. Probiotics alleviate autism-like behaviours in mice. Biology 2013;103;1-3

[72] Messaoudi M et al, 2011, 'Assessment of psychotropic-like properties of a probiotic formulation (Lactobacillus helveticus R0052 and Bifidobacterium longum R0175) in rats and human subjects', *British Journal of Nutrition*, vol. 105, no. 5, pp. 755Nu64.

[73] Tillisch K et al, 2013, 'Consumption of fermented milk product with probiotic modulates brain activity', *Gastroenterology*, vol. 144, no. 7, pp. 1394-1401.

43.8% showed an increase in *Lactobacillus*. The researchers found no statistically significant change in anxiety symptoms among the placebo group.[74]

Gut bacteria can also alter your mood via a set of chemicals called cytokines that have an anti-inflammatory effect in the brain. We know the lining of the healthy digestive tract acts as a barrier. Certain conditions can compromise this wall, inducing leaky gut, and this allows toxic substances and bacterial toxins to enter the bloodstream. In one study, approximately 35% of depressed participants tested positive for leaky gut.[75]

Another study took 124 normal volunteers and showed that those who consumed probiotic-containing yogurt for three weeks had significantly improved moods compared with those who received a placebo.[76]

We now know that depression has an inflammatory component. Some researchers have suggested that the antidepressant effects of certain probiotics might act by altering anti-inflammatory cytokine production in the brain.

Investigators have reviewed many studies that examined the effect of 'psychobiotics' – live organisms that may produce health benefits in patients with disorders of mood and behaviour. When you give a genetically timid and anxious mouse an FMT from a bold mouse, its anxiety and fear completely reverses. When given the probiotic *Bifidobacterium infantis*, a mouse with depressive behaviours resulting from maternal separation completely loses its depressive behaviour. When you pre-treat a mouse with *Lactobacillus rhamnosus*, it seems to stimulate the vagus nerve and prevent depression in mice that have been separated from their mothers. Anxious rats given *Lactobacillus rhamnosus* lose their anxiety and the levels of the calming neurotransmitter GABA go up in their brains. *Lactobacillus helveticus* prevents diet-induced anxiety and *Bifidobacterium longum NCC3001* reverses colitis-induced anxiety in mice.[77]

There is less data for humans, but one study performed on healthy volunteers showed that those who received *Lactobacillus helveticus R0052* plus *Bifidobacterium longum* for 30 days reported significantly lower stress levels than those who received a placebo. In addition, urinary levels of the stress hormone cortisol significantly reduced.[78] Patients with psychotic depression have been shown to respond better to a combination of an antidepressant and the antibiotic

[74] Rao Rayo et al. A randomised, double blind placebo controlled pilot study of a probiotic in emotional symptoms of chronic fatigue. Gut pathology. 209:1-6.

[75] Burke M et al. Acta Psychiatrica Scandinavica 2013; 38-54

[76] Benton D, Williams C, Brown A. Impact of consuming a milk drink containing a probiotic on mood and cognition. Eur J Clin Nutr. 2007;61(3):355-361.

[77] Berick p et al. The anxiolytic effect of Bifidobacterum longum involves vagal pathways for gut brain communication. Neurogastroertoel Motil 2011; 23(12);1132-1139.

[78] Hussain M et al. Mincocycline as an adjunct to for treatment –resistant depression symptoms. Trials 2015; 16:410; Dinan TG & Cryan JF, 2013, 'Melancholic microbes: a link between gut microbiota and depression?' Neurogastroenterol Motil vol. 25, pp. 713-719.

minocycline, suggesting that dysbiotic gut bacteria may be involved in the genesis of depression.

The message is clear. A good gut microbiome is critical to having a happy mood and managing depression.

# Chapter 30

# Gut bacteria and obesity

Stacking on body fat is already a serious problem. Not only for us but, more distressingly, our children. Figures released by the Australian Bureau of Statistics in 2012 confirmed that 60% of Australians are overweight and 25% are classified as medically obese. The burden of obesity in Australia, like most Western countries, is poised to escalate to well over one-third of the population in the next decade. We might even see the incidence of being overweight reaching figures as high as 75%.

Besides being a risk factor for diabetes, heart attack and stroke, obesity has become the number one risk factor for most cancers. It's easily pushing aside tobacco as the number one killer. Aside from obvious triggers like high sugar, high fatty diets and sedentary lifestyles, other factors are coming into play that might help in the fight against obesity-related diseases. Research is uncovering a role for gut bacteria in regulation of body fat.

Evidence, mostly from studies of rodents, suggests that the gut microbiota may play a role in the development of obesity. In obese people, the Firmicutes bacteria are heavily over-represented in the gut at the expense of the *Bacteroides*. We now call the abnormal pattern of gut bacteria in obese people an 'obesogenic microbiome'. This is because evidence points towards alterations in gut bacteria actually causing obesity.[79]

Firmicutes are the kind of gut bacteria that are experts at maximising the absorption of calories from fat and carbohydrates, which is precisely the combination of foods that make up junk food like hamburgers. This becomes a self-fulfilling relationship, as the more fat and carbohydrate you eat, the more Firmicutes proliferate in the gut and more calories they help you absorb from food. The steady growth in obesity is now in train.[80]

Thin people have relatively high proportions of *Bacteroides*, the very bacteria that need fibre from salads and vegetables and fruit. These bacteria actually reduce the caloric salvage from junk foods. The more plant-based food you eat, the more *Bacteroides* you grow in your gut and the more weight you might lose. This is a lean-body human-to-bacteria relationship. Your gut microbiome plays a role in why certain foods make you fat and others make you slim.

---

[79] Conlon MA & Bird AR, 2015, 'The impact of diet and lifestyle on gut microbiota and human health, *Nutrients*, 7(1), pp. 17-44.

[80] Turnbaugh PJ et al, 2008, 'A core gut microbiome in obese and lean twins' [letter], *Nature*, vol. 457, pp. 480-484.

One study found clear differences in the gut microbial communities of obese and lean identical twins. Most notably, the communities from obese twins had less diverse bacterial species. The team took gut microbes from four sets of identical human twins in which one was lean and the other obese. They transplanted faecal microbes from each twin into different groups of germ-free mice (mice with no gut bacteria) and observed the weight and metabolic changes in the mouse groups when they were fed the same diet. Mice populated with microbes from a lean twin stayed slim, whereas those given microbes from an obese twin quickly gained weight and became obese. The 'lean' and 'obese' microbes had different measurable effects on the rodents' metabolism.

As unpleasant as it might seem, mice take great delight in eating each other's poo, so microbiota transfer occurs between cage mates. The researchers decided to place the mice with microbes from lean twins with the obese mice carrying microbes from obese twins. They found that, by eating poo, specific groups of bowel microbes were transferred from lean mice to their obese cage mates who began with less diverse microbial communities. The transfer only occurred in one direction: from lean to obese mice. This transfer appeared to cause the obese mice to lose weight and encourage metabolic profiles resembling those of lean mice.

The researchers were curious about the impact that a typical Western diet, high in refined sugar, saturated fats and low in fibre, would have on these obesity-fighting microbes. The mice had initially been given food that was low in saturated fat and high in fruits and vegetables. The scientists repeated the experiment, but this time fed the mice a diet high in sugar, saturated fats and low in fruits and vegetables. On the Western diet, the mice with 'lean' bacteria weren't able to colonise the mice with 'obese' bacteria, and they stayed obese. These results show that expanding gut microbe diversity can help improve health. However, it takes more than microbes working alone. The success of the approach also depends on a good diet.

To a significant degree, some of us inherit from our parents not only a genetic propensity toward obesity but also a gut microbial population that is skewed towards obesity. What is exciting about these animal experiments is the fact that eating a healthy diet might change the microbiome from an obesogenic one to a microbiome associated with being lean.

Alterations in intestinal microbiota are also associated with insulin resistance, the precursor of diabetes. Another study looked at the effects of faecal transplant of intestinal microbiota from lean human donors to obese male recipients. The control group received transplants of their own microbiome. Six weeks after the infusion of microbiota from lean donors, the insulin sensitivity of the recipients returned to normal, along with increased levels of butyrate-producing intestinal microbiota *Roseburia intestinalis* and *Eubacterium hallii*. It seems that gut microbiota play a role in improving insulin sensitivity in humans. Maybe gut bacteria could be used to prevent diabetes.[81]

We know that certain gut microbes play a role in the control of appetite and satiety. Your gut microbes are dependent on you for food, and as a result they have developed sophisticated ways of controlling your appetite and food choices. Gut bacteria make signal molecules (neuropeptides) that stimulate your own intestine to produce chemical messengers (PYY, GLT1) that make the appetite centre in your brain cause you to be hungry or full.

Beyond affecting your appetite, dysbiotic run on sugars, so they may also be responsible for driving you mad with sweet cravings. No wonder it's so hard to kick the junk food habit when your gut microbes are sending you crazy for sugar. There are no prizes for guessing what probiotic gut bacteria run on: fibre from fruit, salads and vegetables. The next time you feel a craving for sugar, ask yourself who is in charge. Is it you or your gut bacteria? Stand up for yourself![82]

It is not surprising that many of my patients who undergo a microbiome restoration program often report losing weight.

Mrs MP is a 33-year-old nurse who is married with two kids. She suffered with acne rosacea, uterine fibroids but was on no medications. Her major problem was chronic IBS that fluctuated from bouts of chronic diarrhoea with a need to rush to the toilet, tummy cramps, anxiety and flatulence that would alternate with bouts of constipation, bloating and weight gain. This had all started in her 20s after multiple courses of the antibiotic doxycycline that had been prescribed for her acne. All her medical tests were negative and she was told by her doctors that she just had anxiety and an irritable bowel. Probiotics had failed her and she was becoming desperate.

When I saw her she weighed 73.4 kg, with a body mass index (BMI) in the overweight range of 28.5. She underwent a course of FMTs from a lean female donor with a BMI <23. At four months after finishing FMT she reported to have got her life back. She was free of her anxiety and her bowels had returned to normal. An unexpected but pleasing side effect of FMT was that she had lost 6.2 kg in weight. She now weighed 67.2 kg and had a BMI of 26.8.

But changing the gut microbiome can work in reverse too. A now famous case was written up in the medical literature in 2015 illustrating this point. An American doctor from Rhode Island treated a woman for chronic C diff infection with FMT. Unfortunately, he used her overweight daughter as the donor, (which is against current guidelines). Her pre-transplant body weight was 136 lbs with a normal BMI of 26. What happened after receiving her daughter's overweight microbiome was shocking. Just over a year after her FMT, the mother had gained 34 lbs to now weigh 170 lbs with a BMI of 33, which is in the obese range.

[81] Vreize A et al. transfer for the intestinal microbiota from lean donors increase insulin sensitivity in individuals with metabolic syndrome. Gastroenterology 2012; 143; 913-916.

[82] Fetissov S et al. Role of the gut microbiota in host appetite control: bacterial growth to animal feeding behaviour. Nature Reviews Endocrinology 2017; 13:11-25.

Understandably, the doctors put her on a low-calorie diet and exercise program but despite this, at three years from her FMT, she had gained another seven lbs to weigh in at 177 lbs with a BMI of 34.5. This sent shock waves through the medical community, forcing us to take the gut bacteria a bit more seriously.[83]

A healthy microbiota can have significant positive impact on body fat, diabetes, caloric intake and appetite. In other words, you're only as overweight as your gut bacteria will let you be.

---

[83]  N. Alang, C. R. Kelly. Weight Gain After Fecal Microbiota Transplantation. *Open Forum Infectious Diseases*, 2015; DOI: 10.1093/ofid/ofv004

# Chapter 31

# Gut bacteria and rheumatoid arthritis

Rheumatoid arthritis (RA) is a destructive inflammatory autoimmune disease of the joints. The immune system attacks tissues, inflaming joints and damaging organs. Mounting evidence has pointed to a disturbance in the trillions of bacteria that live in the intestines as the potential trigger. Around 1.3 million Americans and 0.5 million Australians have RA.

The condition has a strong genetic component but environmental triggers are known to be involved too. Animal models have demonstrated a clear dysbiotic gut microbiome in RA-prone mice, with overgrowth of *Clostridium* and low levels of *Bifidobacterium* and *Bacteroides*. RA-resistant mice have a different microbiome that is high in the probiotic species Porphyromonadaceae. The RA-prone mice also have abnormal intestinal permeability compared to RA-resistant mice.[84]

Scientists have compared the gut bacteria from faecal samples of patients with RA with those of healthy people. The newly diagnosed and the chronic RA patients had significant gut bacterial dysbiosis compared with healthy people. Various studies have shown the RA type of dysbiosis is characterised by an overgrowth of *Proteus mirabilis*, *Klebsiella pneumoniae* and *Prevotella copri*. RA is also closely linked to an overgrowth of *Porphyromonas gingivalis* in the mouth.[85]

*Porphyromonas gingivalis* in the mouth is a problem for people genetically predisposed to RA because this microbe has an enzyme that converts arginine residues in food into a metabolite called citrulline. Citrulline is highly reactive and binds to many protein peptides in the lining of the mouth and upper digestive tract. Once bound to citrulline, these altered mucosal peptides are seen as foreign and no longer tolerated by the gut immune system. The gut immune system starts pumping out antibodies that attack them, and these antibodies are the most specific biomarkers for RA to date. They are found in 78% of patients with RA.

*Prevotella copri* in the bowel has cell wall antigens that are identical to a collagen that is found in joint cartilage. If cell wall antigens from this microbe get across the leaky gut and into the bloodstream it is likely to lead to the production

---

[84] Gomez A et al, 2012, 'Loss of sex and age driven differences in the gut microbiome characterize arthritis-susceptible 0401 mice but not arthritis-resistant 0402 mice', *PLoS ONE*, vol. 7, no. 4, e36095.

[85] Taneja V, 2014, 'Arthritis susceptibility and the gut microbiome' [letter], *FEBS*, vol. 588, no. 22 pp. 4244–4249.

of antibodies that cross-react with joints, if you are genetically predisposed to RA.[86]

While scientists are debating whether the gut dysbiosis is a result of RA or the cause, we could get on with fixing the dysbiotic microbiome in these patients before they need joint replacements. Having *Porphyromonas gingivalis* in the mouth microbiome and *Prevotella copri* overgrowth and *Bacteroides* undergrowth in the gut microbiome are known risk factors for the development of RA. So why isn't everyone who has a family history of RA having their mouth and gut microbiomes tested for these microbes and, if present, having them eradicated? It's what I do in my practice. And it's what every doctor might do in the future, once they start taking notice of the microbiome.

While there are still no studies looking at the effectiveness of FMT in RA, it has been shown that RA rats given antibiotic treatment to eradicate dysbiotic gut bacteria stopped the progression of the RA.[87]

The story of a New York chef called Seamus Mullen is an illustration of this approach. Mullen was diagnosed with RA in his thirties. After several years of arthritic pains his symptoms became intolerable. Over the next few years he was put on the usual gamut of potent immunosuppressant drugs, which included anti-inflammatory drugs, biologics and steroids, with no luck. Finally, he saw a doctor who suspected his arthritis was driven by an imbalance in his microbiome because of an infection. Mullen followed a strict year-long protocol of exercise, rest, vegetables, fruit and the elimination of refined sugars and grains from his diet. He ate more fermented probiotic foods and took supplements to repair leaky gut and low-level antibiotics to suppress bacterial dysbiosis. He also avoided meat and poultry unless they came from grass-fed animals. After nine months, his blood levels of autoantibodies and inflammatory markers had returned to normal for the first time in a decade, and his RA symptoms had all but disappeared.[88] He is but one case, but one that is worth noting.

In RA, as with all these autoimmune diseases, there are both environmental influences and genetic factors that can induce gut bacterial dysbiosis and alter gut permeability. Addressing these issues should become the focus of any strategy aimed at curing RA along with or part of drug therapy as needed.

---

[86] Brusca S et al, 2014, 'Microbiome and mucosal inflammation as extra-articular triggers for rheumatoid arthritis and autoimmunity', *Current Opinion in Rheumatology*, vol. 26, no. 1, pp. 101-107.

[87] Abdollahi-Roodsaz S et al, 2014, 'Commensal intestinal microbiota drives spontaneous interleukin-1-and T helper 17-mediated arthritis in mice', *Annals of the Rheumatic Diseases*, vol. 73, suppl 1, A87–A88.

[88] Gordinier J, 2011, 'A chef finds healing in food', *The New Yorker*, 2 August.

# Chapter 32

## Gut bacteria and heart disease

Heart disease is the number one killer of people in Western countries. Elevated blood levels of bad (LDL) cholesterol have been associated with cardiovascular disease and early death for several decades. Yet, even with so many people taking cholesterol-lowering drugs, some people are unable to get their cholesterol under control. Could gut bacteria possibly have a role in cardiovascular disease?

Current research has linked gut dysbiosis to heart disease. Certain dysbiotic gut bacteria have been found to metabolise choline and phosphatidyl choline in red meat to release a toxic metabolite that has been linked to the development of cardiac atherosclerosis and heart attack in rats and humans.[89] Supplementation of the probiotic *Lactobacillus plantarum* has been found to reduce the severity of heart attacks by as much as 29%, as well as reducing clotting and LDL cholesterol.[90]

A study in mice found that just seven days of probiotic supplementation with *L. reuteri* reduced their total cholesterol by 38%, bringing their levels close to those of healthy controls.[91] This is better than statin drugs. The probiotic also reduced blood triglycerides by 40% and raised the ratio of beneficial HDL to LDL cholesterol by 20%.

In addition, *L. reuteri*-supplemented mice fed a Western-style diet that contained substantial cholesterol gained significantly less body weight, with lower total and liver fat accumulations, than unsupplemented control mice fed the same diet.[92]

Human studies on *L. reuteri* supplementation have also yielded some impressive results. In one study of adults with elevated cholesterol, subjects consumed either regular yoghurt or one supplemented with *L. reuteri*. Over a six-week period, the supplemented patients' total cholesterol dropped nearly 5% and their LDL cholesterol fell by nearly 9%. Supplemented patients also had a

---

[89] Koeth R et al, 2013, 'Intestinal microbiota metabolism of L-carnitine, a nutrient in red meat, promotes atherosclerosis', *Nature Medicine*, vol. 19, no. 5, pp. 576-585.

[90] Naruszewicz M et al, 2002, 'Effect of Lactobacillus plantarum 299v on cardiovascular disease risk factors in smokers', *American Journal of Clinical Nutrition*, vol. 76, no. 6, pp. 1249-1255.

[91] Taranto MP wt al. evidence for hypocholesterolemic effect of Lactobacillus reuteri in hypercholesteremic mice. J of dairy science 1998;81(9);2336-2360

[92] Fak F et al. Lactobacillus reuteri prevents diet-induced obesity, but not atherosclerosis, in a strain dependent fashion in Apoe-/- mice. PLoS One 2012; 7(10); e46837.

significant decline in concentrations of apolipoprotein B-100 (apoB-100), a known risk factor for cardiovascular disease.[93]

Another study demonstrated similarly impressive results in a group of adults with high cholesterol. After taking *L. reuteri* organisms in capsule form for nine weeks, LDL cholesterol fell by nearly 12%, total cholesterol fell by 9%, non-HDL cholesterol fell by 11%, and apoB-100 fell by 8%. They also had a reduction in their LDL to HDL cholesterol ratio of 13%.[94]

*L. reuteri* appears to lower cholesterol by increasing cholesterol loss from the body through increased cholesterol in stool and increasing cholesterol breakdown in the liver. It secretes an enzyme that traps cholesterol in the intestinal tract and increases signalling to the liver cells to metabolise cholesterol. In this way, *L. reuteri* effectively lowers levels of total and LDL-cholesterol, while driving down inflammation and reducing other metabolic disturbances that raise cardiovascular risks.

Other *Lactobacillus* species fed to obese mice on high-fat diets reduced the pro-inflammatory status of blood vessels, while reducing insulin resistance and blood sugar.[95] These are two major risk factors for heart disease.

Milk fermented with *Lactobacillus plantarum* species lowered glucose, and the inflammatory marker called homocysteine in women with metabolic syndrome, a major cardiovascular risk factor.[96]

When high cholesterol and other lipid disturbances remain unchecked, premature deaths from cardiovascular disease continue to occur despite drug treatments.[97] What if addressing the gut bacteria could change all that?

[93] Jones ML, Martoni CJ, Parent M, Prakash S. Cholesterol-lowering efficacy of a microencapsulated bile salt hydrolase-active Lactobacillus reuteri NCIMB 30242 yoghurt formulation in hypercholesterolaemic adults. British Journal of Nutrition. 2011;9:1-9

[94] Jones M et al, 2012, 'Cholesterol lowering and inhibition of sterol absorption by Lactobacillus reuteri NCIMB: a randomized controlled trial', *European Journal of Clinical Nutrition*, vol. 66, no. 11, pp. 1234-1241.

[95] Chan YK et al. High fat diet induced atherosclerosis is accompanied with low colonic bacterial diversity and altered abundances that correlates with plaque size, plasma A-FABP and cholesterol. BMC Microbiol 2016:16; 264.

[96] Barreto FM et al, 2014, 'Beneficial effects of Lactobacillus plantarum on glycemia and and homocysteine levels in postmenopausal women with metabolic syndrome', *Nutrition*, vol. 30, no. 7-8, pp. 939-942.

[97] Tuohy KM et al, 2014, 'The way to a man's heart is through his gut microbiota – dietary pro-and prebiotics for the management of cardiovascular risk', *Proceedings of the Nutrition Society*, vol. 73, no. 2, pp. 172-185.

# Chapter 33

## Gut bacteria and chronic fatigue

Chronic fatigue syndrome (CFS) is a miserable business. It ruins the lives of those affected and remains poorly understood by medical science. Effective treatments for CFS are all too few. Apart from the relentless fatigue, muscle aches, slow cognition and headaches that define CFS, sufferers are hit with chronic irritable bowel symptoms as well.

Alterations in the intestinal flora have been observed in patients with CFS. The gut dysbiosis found in CFS consists of significant overgrowths of *Prevotella* and the lactate-producing bacteria *Streptococcus* and *Enterococcus* species, accompanied by reduced amounts of the probiotic bacteria *Bifidobacterium* and *E. coli*. The overall degree of biodiversity is reduced, especially within the phylum Firmicutes. This is a proinflammatory gut microbiome.[98]

CFS patients also have a problem with the gut barrier. Blood levels of gut bacterial toxins like lipopolysaccharide and intestinal fatty acid binding protein are elevated. This is evidence of gastrointestinal wall damage, bacteria penetrating through the gut mucus barrier and abnormal permeability.[99]

The persistent fatigue and extreme lack of 'get up and go' has to do with dysfunction of the mitochondria. Mitochondria are the energy furnaces that power our bodies. In the presence of oxygen, they burn glucose and fatty acids to produce the universal molecule of energy called ATP. Energy-packed ATP molecules can travel out of the mitochondria and take their energy anywhere in the body. They are like portable battery packs for the machinery of our body. Mitochondria are present in every cell and are constantly making energy packets to power every thought and movement of our body. Muscle cells have literally hundreds of them.

*Streptococcus* and *Enterococcus* in the intestine convert sugars in our food into lactic acid, the same stuff that is produced by our bodies after very hard exercise. A build-up of lactic acid is what makes you feel so worn out after overdoing it in the gym or running a marathon. We can dispose of L-lactic acid. The problem is D-lactic acid which these bad gut bacteria make in abundance. When you have an overgrowth of *Streptococcus* and *Enterococcus* the load of D-lactic acid in the gut

[98]  Sheedy JR et al, 2009, 'Increased d-lactic acid intestinal bacteria in patients with chronic fatigue syndrome', *In Vivo*, vol. 23, no. 4, pp. 621–628; Frémont M et al, 2013, 'High-throughput 16S rRNA gene sequencing reveals alterations of intestinal microbiota in myalgic encephalomyelitis/chronic fatigue syndrome patients', *Anaerobe*, vol. 22, pp. 50ue6.

[99]  Giloteaux L et al, 2016, 'Reduced diversity and altered composition of the gut microbiome in individuals with myalgic encephalomyelitis/chronic fatigue syndrome', *Microbiome*. vol. 4, p. 30.

is huge and most of it is D-lactic acid, which our bodies have trouble breaking down. D-lactate accumulates in our bodies and damages mitochondria. This is one mechanism that these dysbiotic gut microbes use to reduce our energy supply.

These bacteria also make the gut too acidic. When we eat foods that are high in nitrates, like processed meats, leek, turnip, celery, beetroot, carrot and cabbage, our gut bacteria turn the nitrates in the food into nitrites in the gut. Nitrites are usually passed out in the faeces. When the gut is too acidic, dysbiotic gut bacteria can convert nitrites into nitric oxide and perioxynitrite, which are readily absorbed into the bloodstream. This is a disaster for people with CFS, because they accumulate in the mitochondria and disrupt energy production even more.[100]

Thankfully, this is potentially reversible, but it requires significant cleaning up of the gut dysbiosis aimed at eradicating the bacterial overgrowths of *Streptococcus* and *Enterococcus* and restoring a neutral gut pH. This should be followed by repopulation of the gut with probiotic bacteria, supplementation with nutrients that induce new mitochondrial formation and a specific form of vitamin B12 that scavenges nitric oxide and perioxynitrite from the mitochondria.

Preliminary studies have looked at the use of FMT for CFS. In the first of these, 34 patients with CFS were treated with FMT and followed for many months. Forty-one per cent of patients with CFS reported lasting improvement in their fatigue and 35% showed little or late relief of symptoms.[101]

In 2012, researchers examined a larger cohort of 60 CFS patients who had prominent irritable bowel symptoms and underwent a course of FMT. Seventy per cent responded to FMT treatments and 58% had lasting and complete resolution of their gut and fatigue symptoms over the next 15 to 20 years. These results suggest that FMT may play a role in the treatment of CFS. It is certainly likely to correct the overgrowths of *Streptococcus* and *Enterococcus* that might be drivers of this debilitating condition.

Although FMT has shown promise in some of my patients with IBS and CFS, a lot more work needs to be done in the area – and soon.[102]

One patient was referred to my practice with severe irritable bowel syndrome, which was totally controlling his life and causing him considerable distress. He was having up to 14 bouts of diarrhoea a day with urgency no matter what he took out of his diet. He had become housebound for fear of soiling his pants if he left home for too long and no amount of constipating medications such as Lomotil or Imodium could control it. Not only was his life completely dictated by IBS, but on top of that, he was in constant pain from severe Fibromyalgia and had terrible

---

[100] Brown GC & Borutaite V, 2007, 'Nitric oxide and mitochondrial respiration in the heart', *Cardiovascular Research*, vol. 75, no. 2, pp, 283se90.

[101] Borody TJ, 1995, 'Bacteriotherapy for chronic fatigue syndrome: a long-term followup study', CFS National Consensus Conference.

[102] Borody TJ et al, 2012, 'The GI microbiome and its role in chronic fatigue syndrome: a summary of bacteriotherapy', *Journal of the Australasian College of Nutritional and Environmental Medicine*, vol. 31, no. 3, pp. 3p8.

insomnia. All of which was ruining his life. Over a decade he had consulted multiple doctors, which included gastroenterologists, rheumatologists, naturopaths and integrative health practitioners in a desperate attempt to alleviate his suffering. In the end he turned to FMT despite his doctors telling him that the gut microbiome and faecal transplants were nothing more than 'witch doctoring'. Here is his story in his own words.

Before FMT transplant symptoms:

Life was hell. I was rushing to the toilet between 12-16 times per day. I was hungry all the time, craving sugars and no matter what I ate, I never felt satisfied. My insomnia was out of control. Regularly (approx three or four nights a week) I was awake until 3 or 4 am tossing and turning until finally drifting off for two hours of sleep before my alarm went off at 6 am for work. I was exhausted all the time. I suffered lots of hot flushes both day & night (night times at the worst six to eight times a night which also meant getting out of bed and relieving my bladder).

The terrible muscle and joint aches and fatigue from my fibromyalgia varied throughout the day but I was always in pain. You just learn to ignore it and get on with what you have to do as best you can. The fibromyalgia was worse at night, resulting in two Nurofen caplets three to four nights a week, as a last resort just to get some partial relief from the never-ending pain and get some short bursts of sleep.

This has been going on for 10-12 years. I have seen every doctor and tried every herbal treatment and every medication and been on a very clean, fresh food diet, with no gluten or dairy for over 10 years as well. This helped for a while but I got worse again. My life had become heavily restricted. It was all about resting and finding out where the nearest toilet was. Even doing a food shop I would have to rush to the toilet during that time, sometimes twice. Then, I heard about FMT and decided to investigate it. Dr Froomes was recommended to me through a friend whose relative had been cured by FMT. Here goes nothing.

After the FMT:

I had my first FMT with the colonoscopy on Friday 3rd November 2017. I didn't begin the enemas until the following Thursday due to the Cup weekend. But even after just one FMT, over the weekend my diarrhoea reduced to just four to five motions a day and for the first time they were reasonably firm! Then once the enemas began, within two days, it was a miracle. I was down to two firm motions a day and what's more, for the first time in 12 years, I was sleeping right through the night. I couldn't believe it. After the nine straight days of enemas I continued to have two decent firm motions a day and a bit of wind. I presume that was the colonisation process happening. Occasionally I would have some small fluffy motions that were extra. Two weeks after the treatment was finished I was sleeping soundly all through the night, having two to three formed motions a day. I was eating less, not feeling hungry all the time or craving sugar anymore. I have lost 2½ kg, am down to only two to three short hot flushes a day/night and am able to concentrate more.

But the sweetest thing of all is that fibromyalgia symptoms have quite literally vanished. I still can't believe I'm saying this but I HAVE NO PAIN AT ALL and I have heaps more energy. I am free! I haven't felt this good for approx 15 years. (I had forgotten what it felt like to feel good and energised and normal). I can now go on four to five km walks without worrying where a toilet is, or how much pain I'll have and I also have the energy to do this now. My life has opened up again. I am free from the heavy restrictions of having to know where every toilet is and exhaustion and pain.

I recommend that if you go through with this procedure make sure you stick to the diet because it will really help the FMT to do its job. My normal diet wasn't much different to it so I haven't had trouble sticking to it. Persevere! It's amazing how good the subtle flavour of natural steamed and grilled food is when you get used to it. I have tried an occasional alcoholic drink now that I am past the one-month mark but have found it does affect my bowel so I won't be having any for at least six months.

Thank you, Dr Froomes & the team for providing me with a chance for a new life!

John Thompson (not his real name)

# Chapter 34

# Gut bacteria and multiple sclerosis

Multiple sclerosis (MS) is a devastating autoimmune disease in which the body's own immune system makes antibodies that attack the vital myelin coating of nerves, rendering them useless. Immune-suppressant drugs are still the only proven weapon we have against MS. Most are designed to offset the immune attack on myelin by destroying or regulating immune cells.

Strangely, the MS research community and MS clinicians have not addressed the question of how the myelin-sensitive immune cells keep getting activated. They assume that once these cells are first activated – by a bacterial or viral infection like EBV in childhood, combined with vitamin D deficiency – the autoimmune process just keeps rolling on.

This is very old-school thinking, given what we now know about autoimmune diseases. All the characteristics of MS indicate that the activation of the autoimmune 'attack' cells must be ongoing. Given this, one obvious way of controlling MS is to limit or stop this ongoing activation of the myelin-sensitive immune cells.

Animal and clinical studies have shown that the pathogenesis of MS is associated with the intestinal microbiota. The best explanation is that gut bacterial cell wall antigens from *Methanobrevibacter smithii*, which closely resemble fragments of myelin proteins, pass through the over-permeable gut wall and interact with the immune system. The result is activation of myelin-sensitive immune cells, which churn out antibodies that cross-react with myelin.

The passage of bacterial protein fragments through the gut wall is known to happen with leaky gut. But why is vitamin D deficiency so important? Recent studies have shown that vitamin D is essential to maintaining tight junctions in an intact gut barrier.[103]

There are a number of therapeutic strategies that can help to maintain an intact gut wall. They can also heal the wall if it becomes leaky due to infection or the use of antibiotics. One important strategy is to maintain a dominance of friendly probiotic bacteria in the gut. While a diet that is rich in probiotic foods and oral probiotic supplements is a good place to start, MS patients have to be careful with probiotic yoghurts because some of the milk proteins can be problematic.

---

[103] Juan Kong et al. Novel role of the vitamin D receptor in maintaining the integrity of the intestinal mucosal barrier . 2008. Am J Physiol Gastrointest Liver Physiol 294: G208-G216.

A Swedish study showed that when mice with MS were given three specific strains of *Lactobacillus* their symptoms either stopped or reversed.[104]

In another study, a probiotic was given to five people who had just been diagnosed with relapsing-remitting multiple sclerosis (RRMS). None of the patients had received any other treatments before entering the trial. The volunteers were given the probiotic treatment every two weeks for three months. MRIs checked for the appearance of lesions. The mean number of new lesions dropped from 6.6 at the beginning of the trial to 2.0 at the end. Two months after the probiotic treatment ended, the mean number of lesions climbed to 5.8. The findings suggest the probiotic was beneficial in managing the disease.[105]

Researchers in Sydney have written up three case reports of FMT treatment used to treat constipation-type bowel dysfunction in patients with MS. In all three cases, FMT resulted in significant improvements in bowel function but more surprising was that all three had progressive improvements in their neurological function.[106]

I had one patient who came to my rooms and insisted on trying FMT for her severe MS bowel dysfunction. Together we developed an FMT strategy aimed at resolving her problem. To my surprise, not only did her bowel dysfunction resolve but she also experienced major improvements in her neurological symptoms. Here is her own account of the experience.

> It's very easy to forget what life was like six months ago because I don't ever want to turn back the hands of time. However, the best place to start is at the beginning. I am now 65 and I have lived with MS for 30 years. I believe my journey with MS started at the end of my second pregnancy. I had an abnormal vaginal discharge after delivery and within two weeks of the birth I had a severe *Candida* infection. Four months after the birth I had an episode of optic neuritis. Life went on and I battled with recurring multiple *Candida* infections. Three years later, I had a relapse. I was referred to a neurologist who confirmed the diagnosis of MS.
>
> Over the next 15 years I was relatively unaffected and life was good. But then my condition worsened. I was started on immunosuppressant drugs to slow the progression of the MS. Over the following years my walking reduced, my balance was affected and high-heeled shoes were impossible to wear. It was difficult to write because I found it hard to hold a pen. Using knives was dangerous and standing was only possible for short periods of time. I had times when my symptoms improved a little but it was obvious I was losing the battle.

[104] Lavasani S, Dzhambazov B, Nouri M, Fåk F, Buske S, Molin G, et al. (2010) A Novel Probiotic Mixture Exerts a Therapeutic Effect on Experimental Autoimmune Encephalomyelitis Mediated by IL-10 Producing Regulatory T Cells. PLoS ONE 5(2): https://doi.org/10.1371/journal.pone.0009009

[105] Fleming JO et al, 2011, 'Probiotic helminth administration in relapsing-remitting multiple sclerosis: a phase 1 study', *Multiple Sclerosis*, vol. 17, no. 6, pp. 743ha54.

[106] Borody TJ et al, 2011, 'Fecal microbiota transplantation (FMT) in multiple sclerosis (MS). Am J Gastroenterol, vol. 106, S352.

I discovered FMT after watching a documentary. I was initially repulsed by the idea, but it only took about 20 minutes to become comfortable with the fact that I had to do this. The journey began to find someone who would help me.

Before FMT, I needed a walker for distances more than 50 metres. I exercised in a gravity-free treadmill and with 60% of my weight taken off I was still only able to walk 650 metres at best. I experienced significant foot drop and I had to hold onto walls to stay balanced. I could manage limited work during the day but I suffered extreme fatigue in the evenings. I had severe constipation. It was only possible to open my bowels with laxatives every four to six days.

After FMT, miracles started to happen. My walking improved and I was able to walk confidently for over 600 metres without any aids at all. I could walk 1.2 kilometres on the gravity-free treadmill with only 15% body weight taken off. The fear of falling disappeared as the intensity of the foot drop reduced. I suddenly had lots more energy. I was able to start water aerobics in the evenings twice a week. And best of all I was able to open my bowels every day again.

The improvements were significant and my quality of life was greatly improved. Normality was just around the corner and the finish line was in sight.

It was truly inspiring for me to see the change in her.

Gut dysbiosis and leaky gut appear to be key parts of the MS disease process. It is important to maintain a healthy gut microbial composition and an intact gut barrier to prevent immune activation. Correction of the gut microbiome defects associated with MS could have a positive role for these patients.

Research into the risks and benefits of FMT and probiotics in the prevention and treatment of MS is still in its infancy. However, several lines of evidence indicate that this approach should be taken seriously.

# Chapter 35

# Gut bacteria and Parkinson's disease

Parkinson's disease (PD) causes you to feel that you are so overcome by inertia that you are literally frozen on the spot. It is a progressive neurodegenerative disease in which the parts of the brain that are responsible for smooth, coordinated movement run out of juice and wither away. It leaves people with shakes, rigid limbs, a mask-like face and an inability to walk.

The hallmark of PD is the deposit of a protein-like molecule called alpha-synuclein in the brain. This protein is active and causes dysfunction of nerve structures in the brain. Alpha-synuclein can propagate itself and spread in the brain, causing progressive degeneration of specific brain nervous tissues. There are certain mutations in the alpha-synuclein gene that confer a genetic susceptibility to PD. What causes the onset of the disease is still unknown but, once triggered, the genes produce either an excessive amount or an abnormal form of alpha-synuclein protein.

PD always affects the bowels. More than 80% of sufferers struggle with constipation and this usually predates the onset of PD by several years. What fascinates me is that alpha-synuclein is also found in the colon of almost every PD patient and to a much lesser extent in non-PD colons. In fact, colonic alpha-synuclein is present up to five years before the onset of neurological symptoms. It seems that PD might begin in the gut.[107]

We know that intestinal microbiota interact with the autonomic and the central nervous system via the gut enteric nerves and the vagal nerve. Could alpha-synuclein be a by-product of gut bacterial disturbance and metabolism?

One study examined the intestinal contents of 72 people with PD and 72 without PD. It found that those with PD had levels of *Prevotella* in the gut that were 77.2% lower than the healthy controls. This deficiency of *Prevotella* predicted PD patients with a sensitivity of 86%. An overgrowth of Enterobacteriaceae was associated with more severe postural instability and walking difficulty but less tremor and rigidity.[108]

This is the first evidence that the gut microbiome has a specific pattern of dysbiosis in PD patients and can predict certain patterns of neurological symptoms. *Prevotella* aids in the creation of the B-group vitamins thiamine and folate as well as the maintenance of the intestinal barrier that protects against

---

[107] Shannon KM et al, 2012, 'Is alpha-synuclein in the colon a biomarker for premotor Parkinson's disease? Evidence from 3 cases', *Movement Disorders*, vol. 27, no. 6, pp. 716-719.

[108] Scheperjans F et al, 2015, 'Gut microbiota are related to Parkinson's disease and clinical phenotype', *Movement Disorders*, vol. no. 3, pp. 350-358.

absorption of bacterial and environmental toxins. This finding may therefore have implications not only for diagnosis but also for dietary adjustments or vitamin supplementation for management of PD.

In the future, we hope to be able to properly categorise the specific differences in the gut bacteria that determine the subtypes of PD and manipulate them to alter the course of the disease. In addition, looking for colonic alpha-synuclein may allow us to predict PD before it hits the brain and intervene to prevent the progression of the disease. The gut is much more accessible than the brain, and it can be analysed through colonoscopies and testing of stool samples, so this is very exciting.

# Chapter 36

# Gut bacteria and cancer

Here's a scary thought. Evidence from a wide range of sources suggests that bowel microflora are directly involved in the development of cancer. In fact, the link between gut bacterial-produced carcinogens, inflammation and cancer is so firmly established that the relationship between our gut microbiota and cancer has been termed the 'cancerbiome' or 'oncobiome'. This refers to a particular dysbiotic gut microbiome that is made up of potentially carcinogenic bacteria.

Some human faeces have been shown to be carcinogenic because they contain a number of gene-damaging (genotoxic) substances that have been produced in the bowel by gut bacteria. For example, the intestinal enzyme beta-glucuronidase is involved in releasing a number of dietary carcinogens called cyclic aromatic hydrocarbons from plant glycosides like cycasin.[109]

Another cancerous gut microbe is *Strep gallolyticus*. Studies have shown that up to 80% of people with this bacteria found in their blood already have a bowel cancer or a precancerous colonic polyp.[110] This bacteria has carcinogenic properties that can turn colon cells premalignant and then malignant over time. The authors even go as far as saying that testing for *Strep gallolyticus* could be used as a screening tool to detect people at risk for bowel cancer. I couldn't agree more. Any of my patients that return a stool test positive for *Strep gallolyticus* have a colonoscopy to look for polyps or bowel cancer and then have it eradicated immediately. This is not bacteria you want as part of your gut microbiome. They are a proven carcinogen.

Gut microbiome levels of the butyrate-producing species *Ruminococcus* and *Pseudobutyrivibrio ruminis* are lower in CRC stool specimens, and this correlates with lower gut butyrate levels. Butyrate is the protective fatty acid that provides an energy source that fuels gut repair and the normal functioning of colon cells.

Once again, diet plays a role. When rats are fed a high-meat diet, it switches on the carcinogen-generating enzymes faecal beta-glucuronidase and nitroreductase.[111] But when these rats are given the probiotic *Lactobacillus acidophilus* it significantly decreases the activity of these carcinogenic enzymes.

---

[109] Venturi M et al, 1997, 'Genotoxic activity in human faecal water and the role of bile acids: a study using the alkaline comet assay', *Carcinogenesis*, vol. 18, no. 12, pp. 2353-2359.

[110] Abdulamir et al, 2011, 'The association of *Streptococcus bovis/gallolyticus* with colorectal tumors: the nature and the underlying mechanisms of its etiological role', *Journal of Experimental & Clinical Cancer Research*, vol. 30, no. 1, pp. 11.

[111] Vipperi k et al. Diet, microbiota and dysbiosis: a recipe for colorectal cancer. Food Funct 2016 Apr (4):1731-40.

Just three days of this probiotic was found to inhibit these enzymes and the inhibitory effect lasted for seven days after probiotic dosing ceased.[112]

The World Health Organization has clearly identified diet as a major risk factor for bowel cancer in humans. There is a protective effect of a diet high in fruit and vegetables, and a carcinogenic effect of red meat and processed meats. The much-vaunted apple has been found to be full of antioxidants called phenolic compounds. The extract of apple phenolics has a potent effect on bowel cancer cell lines. It protects colonic cells against carcinogenic DNA damage, improves gut barrier function and inhibits cancer cell invasion. Apples have the potential to block several key stages of the development of bowel cancer. An apple a day is still a great idea as long as you are not badly fructose intolerant.[113]

Another probiotic gut bug, *Lactobacillus johnsonii*, is over-abundant in the gut of mice that are resistant to developing lymphoma. This probiotic can modulate and reduce systemic inflammation and carcinogenicity when given by mouth to lymphoma-prone mice. Given that gut microbiota impact the development of lymphoma, probiotics or FMT might hold promise for reducing lymphoma risk in susceptible individuals. Studies need to be done.[114]

The richness of the gut microbiome is even being looked at in leukaemia treatment. It turns out that the healthier the gut microbiome before stem cell transplant, the less infections people suffer after the transplant and the less graft-versus-host disease they get. While it is unlikely that FMT would be a safe option to repair the gut microbiome after stem cell transplant, it is time to think about nutritional protocols to restore the health of the gut microbiome both before chemotherapy and after stem cell transplant.[115]

It is exciting to think that one day soon we may be able to measure everybody's gut bacterial oncobiome and, if it contains gut carcinogenic bacterial species, we could develop strategies and treatment protocols to change that prognosis. What an incredible step forward in cancer prevention that would be.

Cancer is a diagnosis that evokes innate fear in practically everyone. And the incidence of most cancers continues to escalate. While modern medicine has evolved a plethora of lifesaving strategies for treating many cancers, there are still dramatic failures. Just why some people fail to respond to cancer therapies while others slip easily into remission is still unknown.

[112] Cole CB et al, 1989, 'Effect of probiotic supplements of *Lactobacillus acidophilus* and *Bifidobacterium adolescentis* on ß-glucosidase and ß- glucuronidase activity in the lower gut of rats associated with a human faecal flora', *Microbial Ecology in Health and Disease*, vol. 2, no. 3, pp. 223 225.

[113] McCann MJ et al, 2007, 'Anti-cancer properties of phenolics from apple waste on colon carcinogenesis in vitro', *Food and Chemical Toxicology*, vol. 45, no. 7, pp. 1224mic30.

[114] Yamamoto ML et al, 2013, 'Intestinal bacteria modify lymphoma incidence and latency by affecting systemic inflammatory state, oxidative stress, and leukocyte genotoxicity', *Cancer Research*, vol. 73, no. 14, pp. 4222e4232.

[115] Taur Y et al, 2015, 'Role of intestinal microbiota in transplantation outcomes', *Best Practice and Research Clinical Haematology*, vol. 28, no. 2-3, pp. 155ol61.

New research is pointing the finger at the gut microbiome as one very real variable that determines how well your body is going to respond to certain cancer treatments. In other words, your gut microbiome might be the reason your cancer therapy will or will not cure you.

Immunotherapy of the aggressive skin cancer known as malignant melanoma has saved many lives. This clever form of treatment can switch on the white blood cells of your own immune system to seek out and destroy melanoma cancer cells like cancer-seeking missiles.

Researchers from the prestigious MD Anderson Cancer Center in Texas discovered that a good gut microbiome (biodiversity), particularly one that was rich in Clostridiales, Ruminococcaceae and Faecalibacterium, significantly prolonged progression-free survival after immunotherapy for melanoma compared to patients with different gut microbes. It turns out that these particular afore-mentioned probiotic gut bacteria stimulated the immune response of the melanoma patients to a much greater extent when given immunotherapy. So, they were better equipped to mount a truly effective immune-mediated attack on the melanoma cancer cells.

What the researchers did next was even more exciting. They looked for a causal link between a favourable gut microbiome and response to immune checkpoint blockade by giving faecal transplants from humans with melanoma, who were either responsive to immunotherapy or had failed to respond to immunotherapy, into germ-free mice with melanoma. Okay, that's a mouthful but the results are worth reading on.

The melanoma mice that got FMTs from humans who were responsive to immunotherapy therapy had a significant reduction in melanoma tumour growth. Whereas the mice who got FMTs from humans who failed immunotherapy had a lot more aggressive tumour growth.

The mice that got FMTs from humans who were responsive to immunotherapy therapy also showed lots more Faecalibacterium in their mouse poo and responded beautifully to immunotherapy therapy. Whereas the others failed to respond to immunotherapy.

The responsive FMT mice showed loads more tumour-killing white cells in the blood, the gut and the spleen. And the melanoma tumour deposits became packed with significantly more tumour-killing white cells. Which suggests that the new gut microbes boosted the immune system response to immunotherapy to such a degree that the tumours became 'hot' with immune attack cells. A melanoma deposit becomes 'hot' when immunotherapy stimulates the person's immune system to swarm into the tumour, effectively lighting it up, with attack cells. When this happens, the melanoma is destroyed and the cancer disappears.

These remarkable results are the first to indicate the gut microbiome modulates responses to melanoma immunotherapy in melanoma mice and human patients. It is beginning to look like a favourable gut microbiome, that means one that is diverse and enriched with a high relative abundance Ruminococcaceae and

Faecalibacterium will most likely determine whether a person will cure melanoma with immunotherapy or not. And it does so by enhancing the tumour-killing arms of the immune system throughout the body and in the microenvironment of the tumour deposits themselves. Awesome.

In contrast, patients and mice with an unfavourable gut microbiome, which is one that is not rich and is low in Ruminococcaceae and Faecalibacterium but high in Bacteroidales, have reduced systemic and anti-tumour immune capabilities in response to immunotherapy. Which means it fails.[115.2]

In the future, it's likely that we will consider preconditioning cancer patients' gut microbiomes prior to treatment to ensure they get cured with the proposed immunotherapy.

---

[115.2] Gopalakrishnan V et al. Gut micro biome modulates response to anti-PD-1 immunotherapy inmelanoma patients. Science 2017. 10.1126 University of Texas MD Anderson.

# Chapter 37

# Gut Bacteria & Autism Spectrum Disorder

Some may consider it strange, absurd even, but Autism Spectrum Disorder or (ASD) may turn out to be caused by an unhealthy gut microbiome. Well, I don't find it strange at all given that there is continuous communication between the bacteria that reside in a child's gut, their developing brain, and their immune system. In fact, it seems highly probable.

Recent studies suggest that autism may even be triggered before birth. This hypothesis derives from a study that found pregnant mice with inflammatory gut microbiomes gave birth to baby mice (pups) that displayed autistic social and communicative behaviour.[116]

Consider even further that the conduit of a pregnant mother's stress induced inflammation to a developing child's brain might be through the gut microbiome? The answer is an emphatic yes! When researchers from the University of Pennsylvania Medical School subjected pregnant mice to continuous psychological stress it significantly increased the risk of autism behaviour in their offspring.

Even more defining was the finding that the composition of the vaginal flora of the stressed mothers showed a significant loss of several critical probiotic bacterial species such as Lactobacillus and became dysbiotic. This unhealthy vaginal microbial zoo was then passed on to the newborn mice during the vaginal delivery. The newborn mice pups all displayed autism behaviours. They also found the unhealthy mice pup gut flora reduced their ability to absorb specific brain nutrients from food and in turn this impaired brain development. The most severely affected region of the newborn's brain was the hypothalamus, which is mainly associated with stress responses.[117]

The researchers concluded that the mother's microbiome appears to exert inflammatory responses that alter both the gut flora and the developmental behaviour of their offspring. This effect is likely due to the inflammatory by-products produced by harmful bacteria in the mother's gut, which are absorbed into the maternal blood stream and transferred to the developing foetus via the placenta or the amniotic fluid. These inflammatory bacterial 'toxins' can therefore begin to disrupt normal brain development and function in utero.

---

[116] Catherine R. Lammert et al. Cutting Edge: Critical Roles for Microbiota-Mediated Regulation of the Immune System in a Prenatal Immune Activation Model of Autism. The Journal of Immunology. 1 July 2, 2018, ji1701755.

[117] Howerton C & Bale T. Prenatal programming: At the intersection of maternal stress and immune activation. Horm Behav. 2012 August ; 62(3): 237-242.

So having been condemned to autism in utero, is it game over for the developing child? No it's not. Childbirth forms only part of the explanation. Inheriting what I term a 'pro-ASD gut microbiome' during childbirth might set abnormal brain development and behaviours in motion but they won't continue to manifest unless the developing child continues to harbour and foster these same bad gut bacteria. The implication? There is ample time to intervene to transform the child's dysbiotic microbiome into a probiotic gut microbiome, that is, one that will allow normal brain and behavioural development.

After birth, a dysbiotic gut microbiome can continue to damage and disrupt normal brain and behavioural development. Children with Autism Spectrum Disorder (ASD) invariably have chronic bowel problems. It's not surprising that the major factor associated with these gastrointestinal (GI) issues in ASD kids is an unhealthy mix of resident gut flora or dysbiosis. Studies comparing the make-up of the gut microbiome of children with ASD, when compared with their non-ASD peers, have shown global reductions in the amount of good, probiotic gut bacteria, with particular deficits in Lactobacillus and Bifidobacteria levels [118] coupled with a striking overgrowth of bad Clostridial bacteria.[119]

Researchers at Arizona State University also found significant differences in the levels of 50 different metabolites produced by gut bacteria in kids with ASD compared with the control group. The study found that certain by-products of bacterial fermentation in the bowel, such as propionic acid, which are produced by dysbiotic bacteria like Clostridia and Desulfovibrio, interfere with brain development and behaviour in children.

Feeding non-ASD mouse pups a diet high in propionic acid from birth caused intestinal inflammation and the development of autism behaviours. Abnormal blood levels of chemicals known as acylcarnitines, which are related to propionic acid production, have also been found in autistic children. This abnormal oxidation of fatty acids has been shown to cause dysfunction of the mitochondrial energy factories in autistic children.[120]

It was first shown 18 years ago that 8 out of 10 children with slower onset autism showed significant improvements in behaviour and socialisation when treated with an antibiotic called vancomycin which kills *Clostridium* and Desulfovibrio.[121] Follow-up research in this area had been scarce until in 2017 it was re-examined with stunning results. Changing the gut flora of children with ASD using faecal microbiota transplant (FMT) caused significant and sustained

[118] Ding HT et al. Gut Microbiota and Autism: Key Concepts and Findings. J Autism Dev Disord. 2017 Feb; 47(2):480-489.

[119] Finegold et al. Gastrointestinal Microflora Studies in Late-Onset Autism. Clinical Infectious Diseases 2002; 35(Suppl 1):S6-16.

[120] Frye RE et al. Unique acyl-carnitine profiles are potential biomarkers for acquired mitochondrial disease in autism spectrum disorder. Transl Psychiatry (2013) 3, e220.

[121] Sandler RH et al. Short-term benefit from oral vancomycin treatment of regressive-onset autism. J Child Neurol 2000 Jul;15(7):429-35.

improvements in both bowel problems and ASD-related socialisation and behaviour.

Let's take a closer look at this. Researchers at Ohio State University looked at 18 kids with both ASD and chronic irritable bowel symptoms. They were given two weeks of the antibiotic vancomycin followed by eight weeks of daily FMTs. After 16 weeks they noticed two startling results. Firstly, the gut symptoms of the kids reduced by 82%, and secondly the ASD-related symptoms improved significantly. The improvements continued for the full eight weeks after FMT stopped. They assessed the social and behavioural improvements in the children using both the Parent Global Impressions-III (PGI-III) assessment and the doctors' Childhood Autism Rating Scale (CARS). The research also found a direct inverse correlation between the severity of the bowel symptoms and autism behaviour. The more pronounced the bowel symptoms, the more apparent the autism behaviours.[122]

While things are definitely moving in the right direction regarding the research into the relationship between ASDs and the gut microbiome, it remains slow and more urgent work is needed.

I had one mother consult me about her seven-year-old boy after she had read about FMT helping autistic children in the online medical literature. Let's call him Adam (not his real name). Adam was born with cerebral palsy classified as Gross Motor Function Classification System Level 2. This means he can walk in most settings and climb stairs holding onto a railing. He may experience difficulty jumping, running or walking long distances and balancing on uneven terrain, inclines, in crowded areas or in confined spaces.

Adam was also diagnosed with severe autism described as Level 2 under the Autism Spectrum Disorder 299.00 (F84.0) DSM-V, American Psychiatric Association, 2013 classification. This meant that Adam required 'substantial support due to marked deficits in verbal and nonverbal social communication skills; social impairments apparent even with supports in place; limited initiation of social interactions; and reduced or abnormal responses to social overtures from others.'

Parents of autistic kids are incredible people. They are patient and loving with their children and tirelessly dedicated to helping them. They are also often better researched than most doctors! At the initiation of his mum, Adam had a course of the antibiotic vancomycin followed by faecal microbial transplants. Here is Adam's story as described by his mother.

> Adam did the FMT program easily without really being bothered by it. We didn't tell anyone we were doing the FMTs because we were concerned that his teachers and therapists would be looking for changes in order to report something back to us. This meant they were blinded to the treatment.

---

[122] Kang et al. Microbiota Transfer Therapy alters gut ecosystem and improves gastrointestinal and autism symptoms: Microbiome (2017) 5:10.

After only the second FMT, I received an email from Josh's teacher reporting that he had been very focused at school and was concentrating for much longer periods at a time. At this point I still didn't tell her about the treatment.

From then on, each day at school pick-up, for about a week, his teacher reported more and more improvements that were obvious to her – better concentration, improvement in comprehension, more interested in what his peers were doing. Even though he wasn't engaging with them in a typical manner, he was still approaching them and looking over their shoulder to see what they were doing. At the end of the week, she couldn't help but ask me if we had been doing anything differently because she said the changes were very obvious and happening all in a short period of time.

His teacher also told me that the kids in his class noticed the changes. A couple of the boys approached her during 'free time' in the classroom and they were very excited. Apparently Adam had gone over to them and called them both by name and asked them what they were doing. Admittedly he would have been attracted by the fact that they were playing on their iPads (his favourite thing), but the fact that he had called them by name was what excited the boys who said "we didn't think he even knew our names".

This was especially important to me as I feel like Adam has always known exactly what is happening around him and who people are; he just doesn't have the interest factor to acknowledge or engage, and I feel like FMT has improved this.

A couple of weeks after the FMT, Adam's physio asked me if we had done anything differently because she noticed much more focus during her sessions (her sessions are all functional), and a lot of independence or attempts at independence. He finally seemed to want to do his therapy and achieve the goals rather than go through the motions and just do it because he is agreeable by nature.

My husband, aware that we were doing FMTs, was away for work at the time of the FMTs and when he came home about a week after completion, he too noticed that Adam's interaction and speech had both improved.

Overall, we have seen a marked improvement in Adam's social skills – he doesn't have the language to reflect how far he has come, but it's obvious to everyone that knows him. He will say hello to people and is very interested in who people are. He will say, "Hello, what's your name please?" Which is a taught phrase but now he says it of his own volition and because he genuinely wants to know.

After the FMTs I noticed Adam is also very engaged when in the car. He looks out the window and sometimes comments on what he sees – this has never happened before.

An example: We were in the car waiting at traffic lights and traffic was stopped because of an oncoming ambulance which had its lights and sirens on. We said to our non-autistic three-year-old daughter who could hear the sirens, "Chloe, what do you think it's going to be?" (meaning police, fire, ambos), and she yelled out "ambulance". At the same time Adam yelled out "police car!" We were gob smacked because he DOES NOT show interest in anything like this at all. This is a little game we play with Chloe all the time because she loves the sirens and emergency vehicles, and in all the times we've done it Adam has never engaged. I'm sure many people would put this down to coincidence/growth/ maturity etc, but there are too many little examples like this that happened so close to the FMT for this to be the case.

He is also sleeping better. Before FMTs he would lie awake for hours at a time in the night and couldn't get to sleep no matter how hard he tried. He always had purple rings under his eyes and looked fatigued. But since having the FMTs he is sleeping well through the night again and those purple rings under his eyes have gone.

We have seen some improvement in his speech also. He is still nowhere near his peers, however due to his severe language delay (expressive worse than receptive) improvement in speech really wasn't expected at all. That said, Adam has started to expand his language from just using enough words strung together to get by, to using meaningful sentences. One example is:

Pre FMT: "I need a drink with ice please" (a taught phrase that he says the exact same way every time).

Post FMT: "I'm thirsty, I need a drink with ice please."

The most amazing achievement though is his ability to identify emotions. This is something that we, and the therapists, have been working on for years, with no improvement. My husband is away a lot for work and Adam never verbalises how he is feeling about this. He is very close to his dad though, so we have always wondered if it bothered him. On the most recent trip away, I was putting Adam to bed and he started to cry and said, "I miss Daddy." The next night he said, "I'm feeling sad because I miss Daddy." I wasn't sure if I was heartbroken for him or excited by his expressing of emotion!

When my husband returned home late on a Sunday night, they didn't get to spend much time together and then my husband took him to school the next day. When he left the classroom Adam became very distressed and was crying. He had a conversation with his teacher.

Teacher: "How are you, Adam?"

Adam: "I'm upset."

Teacher: "Why are you upset?"

Adam: "Because I want to be with Daddy."

The reason this is so profound is because Adam has been taught the appropriate response to the question "How are you?" Every time, without fail, he says "I'm great" and he will say this through tears, if he's angry, if he's happy – it's always the same response. His teacher was so shocked with the exchange that she emailed me straight away – both sad for Adam and happy with the ability to recognise how he was feeling.

This has also extended to his sister and Adam is now noticing how she is feeling too. He will ask, "Chloe, are you happy?" if she is crying or yelling.

Sometimes he will say to me, "Is Chloe happy?" What's interesting about that is that he has never before even indicated that he can hear her yelling or crying even though she is sitting right next to him.

I'm not suggesting that FMT is the magic bullet that has made all these sudden changes in Adam. However, the changes all occurred within a short period of FMT, and I feel like even if it wasn't the FMT that caused these leaps forward in his development, it was the catalyst to allow it happen and allow him to unlock all these new skills.

The graphs on the following page illustrate how Adam's gut microbiome changed after FMT therapy. Following FMT, the most striking changes were the increases in the phylotype Firmicutes, which contain the probiotic Lactobacillus, and the phylotype Actinobacteria, which contain the probiotic Bifidobacterium, both of which have been described as lacking in autistic children.

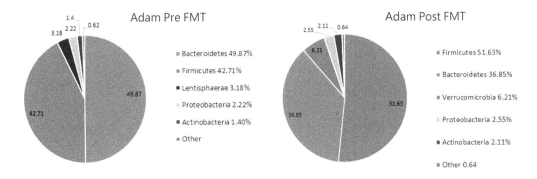

Could autism one day be treated or even prevented with therapies designed to restore a healthy gut microbial balance in the pregnant mother and her newborn baby? I know so! But let's expedite the researching now.

# Section 3

# How to fix your gut

# Chapter 38

## You are what your gut eats

Using a specific program of gut cleansing, dietary modification and symbiotic supplements, you can begin the process of engineering a strong gut microbiome that will improve your health, wellbeing, digestion, nutritional state, brain function and mood. All this will start you on the road to recovering from irritable bowel, IBD, obesity and autoimmune diseases.

The gut reload process has two critical phases: removing toxic gut bacteria and their biofilms, followed by reloading with good gut bacteria. This can all be done naturally, using plant extracts, specific nutrients and natural prebiotic and probiotic foods.

But first you need to understand one very important fact. What is casually referred to as 'food' is absolutely nothing of the sort. You will have heard the expression 'You are what you eat', but the reality is that 'Your gut bacteria are what you eat'.

For example, probiotic bacteria feed on soluble fibre from fresh salads, fish, fruits, nuts, seeds and vegetables, and they produce vitamins, minerals and short-chain fatty acids that are necessary for life. Dysbiotic bacteria feed on sugar, fructose and other types of refined carbohydrates that are found in processed white flour, bread, lollies, chocolate, cakes, pastries, biscuits, soft drinks, corn chips, potato chips, packaged foods, sauces, ice-cream, jam and white rice, and they produce lactic acids, aldehydes and toxic gases. Then there are yeasts that feed on simple sugars that are found in almost all processed and packaged foods. They ferment these sugars to produce a host of toxic chemicals called volatile organic compounds that are similar to alcohols and aldehydes. These chemicals often give rise to leaky gut, brain fog and fatty liver. You get the idea!

Diet plays a significant role in determining the make-up of the gut microbiota. And what we eat these days would not have been classified as food by any human or probiotic gut bacteria that might come in contact with it in the previous 2.5 million years of our coevolution.

Take a look at the ingredients of a packet of savoury biscuits: Wheat Flour, Vegetable Oil, Cheese (Contains Milk), Sesame Seeds, Salt, Vegetable Extract (From Maize), Yeast, Tomato Powder, Spices, Glucose, Raising Agent (E500), Natural Flavour, Starch, Onion Powder, Artificial Colours (Turmeric, Cochineal), Emulsifier (E322), Antioxidant (E306), Antioxidant (E304).

Or a cup of top-selling powdered soup: Noodles (34%) (Wheat Flour, Artificial Colour [Carotene]), Vegetables (Onion [25%], Red Capsicum [2%]), Maize (corn) Starch, Creamer, Vegetable Oil (Contains Soybean Derivative), Glucose Syrup, Milk Protein, Mineral Salts (339, 450), Fish Sauce (3%), Maltodextrin (From

Wheat), Flavour Enhancer (621), Favour Enhancer (635), Sugar, Mineral Salt (Potassium Chloride), Salt (Sodium Chloride), Flavours (Contain Wheat, Milk, Soybean Derivatives), Parsley (0.5%), Hydrolysed Corn Protein, Vegetable Oils (Sunflower, Soybean), Colours (Carotene, Caramel lV, Carmine), Food Acid (Citric), Chilli, Lemongrass Extract.

Or a popular chocolate biscuit: Sugar, Wheat Flour, Vegetable Oil, Milk Solids, Cocoa Butter, Cocoa Mass, Golden Syrup, Colours (E150C [From Wheat], E129, E110, E133, E102), Cocoa Emulsifiers (E322] From Soy), E476), Salt Raising Agent (E500), Flavours. Contains Milk Chocolate 38%.

These ingredients read more like a chemistry experiment than a food recipe. It's frightening. And yet these processed 'food-equivalents', as I call them, are sold to us as food by the ton. The number one ingredient in all these so-called foods is highly refined wheat flour plus cornstarch, followed closely by refined sugar.

Refined flours are treated just like sugar by our bodies. Wheat flour comes from wheat and cornstarch comes from corn, but the nutrient-rich and fibre-dense outside husks are stripped away. All that remains is the nutrient-depleted endosperm, which is then ground up into fine flour. Wheat flour gives food consistency, mouthfeel and taste, and cornstarch is used in processed foods to thicken them. Cornstarch is used in baked goods and fried foods and is considered gluten-free. It is also used in the manufacturing of bioplastics due to its anti-stick properties.

The modern Western diet is dominated by factory-processed chemical mixtures that are completely devoid of any nutritional value. Clever packaging and advertising is designed to trick consumers into thinking they contain the goodness of natural wholefoods. These food-like substances are mass produced, sugar-laden, antibiotic chemical mixtures that are passed off as food because they taste extremely good and have a colourful photograph of real wholefood on their packaging. In reality, they contain almost no natural food nutrients. They are chemical mixtures dreamed up by food scientists who are experts in chemicals, not nutritionists or dieticians.

Yet we still expect our gut bacteria to be rich, plentiful and entirely composed of healthy probiotic bacteria that will provide significant health benefits. Instead we and our gut bacteria become nutrient-deficient and this has disastrous results for our health.

# Chapter 39

# The problem with wheat

We are not genetically evolved to eat grass seeds like wheat, rye and barley. Our genes haven't changed significantly in the last 4000 years, much less the last 10,000 or two million. And, regardless of our ethnicity or any ideology that we might happen to have, we are all fundamentally hunter-gatherers. That's how we and our gut microbiota have coevolved for 2.5 million years. And, as the medical anthropologist Boyd Eaton has stated, 99.99% of our genes were formed before the development of agriculture. We have only been eating wheat for 200-500 generations, which isn't enough time for our genes to adapt to completely digest a new food.

The first problem with wheat is that our digestive juices and enzymes can't properly break down gluten, the protein component of wheat. Gluten is full of disulfide bonds. Disulfide bonds are so tough that they are used to make super-tough vulcanised rubber.

Some intestinal bacteria can break down some of those disulfide bonds. Partially broken-down gluten proteins, called gluten peptides, can be absorbed into the blood but they trigger an immune response from the gut and the body. Gluten peptides cause abnormal permeability. They bind a zonulin receptor on the surface of the intestinal cells and stimulate them to produce zonulin. Zonulin disrupts and opens up tight junctions and the result is leaky gut. This effect on gut permeability lasts for several hours after eating gluten. If gluten is eaten at every meal, the leaky gut lasts all day.

The second problem with wheat is that our bodies break down its carbohydrate components into sugar. Have you ever taken a bite of white bread and left it in your mouth? Pretty soon the neutral taste of the bread is replaced by a sugar-like sweetness. That's because the enzyme called amylase in your saliva is breaking down the bread into sugars.

Refined white wheat flour has had every beneficial nutrient that nature gave it processed out. What is left is mostly carbohydrate and some gluten. The carbohydrate component of bread is nothing more than long chains of sugar joined together like beads on a necklace. That's fine if there's a famine but it's extremely bad for our health if there is already more than enough fat and protein in our diet.

Carbohydrate-containing foods are rated on a scale called the glycaemic index (GI). This scale ranks foods based on how high and how quickly they elevate your blood sugar levels two hours after eating them. The most potent food is pure sugar and it has the highest-possible GI score of 100. Other carbohydrates, like oats, are broken down more slowly and release their sugar content into the bloodstream more gradually. They have low glycaemic indexes (GI less than 55). Low GI foods prolong digestion and help us feel full. Good old white bread has a GI score of 100. Your body sees bread exactly the same as eating pure sugar.

It's very damaging to the body to have a high blood sugar level for any period of time. Firstly, the sugar molecules in blood stick to our own tissue proteins and form damaging molecules called advance glycation end (AGE) products. AGEs damage tiny blood vessels in our kidneys, heart and brain. This is why diabetics get kidney failure, heart attacks and strokes. Secondly, the rapid and very high rise in blood sugar from eating wheat flour causes a surge in insulin. The insulin removes the sugar from our bloodstream before it can do too much damage. It literally pumps sugar into fat cells for storage, which leads directly to obesity. Thirdly, sugar feeds bad gut bacteria. The sugars contained in food made from white wheat flour encourage overgrowth of dysbiotic bacteria in the small and the large bowel. It is one of the causes of gut bacterial dysbiosis.

The third problem with wheat is that it has evolved its own defence against predators. It contains a lectin called wheat germ agglutin (WGA). Lectins are a type of protein that can bind to cell membranes and they are small enough to pass through the gut barrier and into the body.[123] Even in tiny doses, lectins can be fatal if inhaled or injected directly into the bloodstream.

WGA starts its attack by damaging the gut. It binds to carbohydrate molecules on the surface of the delicate cells that line the intestine, causing shedding. This reduces the total surface area that is available for the absorption of nutrients. WGA is quite proinflammatory. It stimulates the synthesis of cytokines (pro-inflammatory chemical messengers) in intestinal and immune cells and has been shown to play a causative role in patients with chronic gut inflammation. Anti-WGA antibodies in human blood cross-react with other proteins, indicating that WGA may contribute to autoimmunity. WGA also appears to play a role in the pathogenesis of coeliac disease that is entirely distinct from that of gluten. In addition, WGA is thought to be capable of inhibiting nerve growth factors and it has an insulin-like action, which means it may contribute to weight gain and insulin resistance.[124]

When we consume glucosamine supplements, WGA binds to the pulverised chitin in the glucosamine supplements instead of to our own cells, sparing us from its inflammatory impact. Many millions of people who have greatly reduced their pain and suffering by taking glucosamine and NSAIDs might be better to remove wheat from their diets.

[123] Ji S, 2008, '200 dark side of wheat', *GreenMedinfo*, <http://www.greenmedinfo.com/page/dark-side-wheat-new-perspectives-coeliac-disease-wheat-intolerance-sayer-ji>, viewed 28 June 2017.
[124] Ji S, 2008, op. cit.

# Chapter 40

## The problem with emulsifiers

Some of the most frequently used food chemicals are emulsifiers. What are emulsifiers? When you add oil to water, the oil sinks to the bottom and the lighter water sits on top. Emulsifiers are molecules with one water-loving (hydrophilic) end and one oil-loving (hydrophobic) end. They make it possible for water and oil to mix together nicely, creating a smooth emulsion.

Emulsifiers are added to bread to strengthen it, increase its volume, give breadcrumbs a softer feel and increase shelf life. Emulsifiers give chocolate its silky consistency and allow it to be moulded into any shape. They add textural smoothness to ice-cream, frozen yoghurt and mousse and stop them melting too easily after serving. They give margarine its stability, texture and taste and allow the fats in processed meat to be distributed evenly to give them a rich mouthfeel. Emulsifiers are very hard to avoid unless you make your own food.

Although they are approved for human consumption and are a ubiquitous component of processed foods, emulsifiers should not be eaten. They are detergent-like chemicals and they strip away the protective gut lining and cause abnormal gut permeability. They have been shown to increase bacterial translocation across the gut wall and promote IBD.

A 2015 study tested the safety of two of the most commonly used emulsifiers in mice. They fed the mice relatively low concentrations of these emulsifiers and found to their horror that they induced inflammation, obesity and metabolic syndrome. And when they fed emulsifiers to mice that were genetically predisposed to IBD, the mice rapidly developed severe colitis. When the researchers looked at the gut of the mice with emulsifier-induced metabolic syndrome, high blood sugar and obesity, they saw that gut bacteria composition had changed. The protective gut mucous layers had been stripped away, allowing bacteria to come in direct contact with the cells lining the gut, and there were increased inflammatory cells in the gut wall as a result. The researchers concluded that these common food additives may promote ulcerative colitis and Crohn's disease as well as metabolic syndrome.

Microbiologist Benoit Chassaing said the effects seen in mice 'may be observed in humans as well'. The incidence of inflammatory bowel disease and metabolic syndrome started rising in the middle of the 20th century – roughly the same time that food manufacturers began widespread emulsifier use. 'We were thinking there was some non-genetic factor out there, some environmental factor, that would be explaining the increase in these chronic inflammatory diseases,' said immunologist Andrew Gewirtz.[125] The researchers are planning human studies and are already studying other emulsifiers.

---

[125]  Chassaing B et al, 2015, Dietary emulsifiers impact the mouse gut microbiota promoting colitis and metabolic syndrome', *Nature*, vol. 519, no. 7541, pp. 92-96.

# Chapter 41

## Fibre, starch and FODMAPs

Fibre, starch and FODMAPs are all different types of carbohydrates. Learning about them will help you to restore a healthy gut microbiome.

Dietary fibre is an essential healthy type of carbohydrate. Fibre is the indigestible portion of the plants we eat. We can't digest it, so it goes through the gut largely unaltered and helps form stools that are very satisfying to pass. These indigestible plant fibres are actually food for our gut bacteria. Fibre contains vitamins and nutrients that healthy probiotic bacteria need and keeps them happy and well fed. Probiotic gut bacteria also use fibre to produce fuel for our intestinal cells. Fibre is low in calories and is a low GI food. Even though it is poorly absorbed it rarely triggers gut symptoms because the bacterial fermentation of plant fibre is slow. Gas production is not fast enough to create much gaseous distension. Of course, eating too much fibre may cause symptoms in some people.

Complex starches are long chains of simple sugars that are strung together to form carbohydrate chains, like those found in peas, oats and beans. The body can digest them to yield vitamins, nutrients and sugars. Because complex starches take a while to digest, they are also considered low GI foods and are unlikely to cause gut problems in most people. But beware, some of the complex starchy foods like legumes also contain high levels of FODMAPs and therefore may aggravate IBS in FODMAP-sensitive people.

Refined starches are made by refining complex wholegrain starches. The healthy fibre, nutrients and vitamins contained in the germ and bran are stripped away. This is how we get white flour and cornstarch, which are used to make white bread, cakes, pastries and pasta. When eaten, these refined starches take on the properties of simple sugars and are processed in the same way as sugar by the body. They are high GI foods that foster overgrowth of dysbiotic gut bacteria.

FODMAPs is an acronym for 'fermentable oligosaccharides, disaccharides, monosaccharides and polyols'. The simplest way to understand FODMAPs is to think of them all as a type of carbohydrate that is found in the food we eat.

'Fermentable' means that they are fermented in the large intestine by colonic bacteria, which produces gas and fatty acids that can cause diarrhoea, wind and bloating.

Oligosaccharides, disaccharides, monosaccharides and polyols are all carbohydrates, or sugars. Oligosaccharides are medium-length chains of sugar units, such as fructans and galacto-oligosaccharide (GOS). Fructans are found primarily in wheat, rye, garlic and onions. GOS is found in legumes like lentils and chickpeas. In order for oligosaccharides to be digested and absorbed they need to be broken down, but there is no human enzyme that can cleave the bonds.

Fructans and GOS are poorly absorbed by everyone. Disaccharides are small carbohydrates made up of two simple sugars joined together. Lactose is the disaccharide that is found in cow's milk. Lactose must be split into single sugar molecules, or monosaccharides, by the enzyme lactase in order to be absorbed. Some people can have deficiencies in lactase production, resulting in malabsorption of lactose which can act as an IBS trigger. Sucrose is also a disaccharide. It requires an enzyme called sucrase to break it down into monosaccharides for absorption.

Monosaccharides are single sugar molecules that can be readily absorbed by the small intestine. Monosaccharides include fructose, which is found in fruits like apples and pears as well as in honey.

Polyols, or sugar alcohols, such as sorbitol and mannitol occur naturally in some fruits and vegetables. They are also manufactured for use as artificial sweeteners. They are much lower in calories than glucose but taste almost as sweet. You see them in 'sugar free' or 'artificially sweetened' products and if you look closely you will notice the packs contain warnings about excess consumption and possible diarrhoea. The term FODMAPs is a way of grouping together specific simple carbohydrates, or small sugars, that can be poorly absorbed and rapidly fermented by bacteria in the bowel. The reason IBS sufferers respond so poorly to FODMAPs is that these sugars are dumped into the large bowel where trillions of bacteria ferment them. Dysbiotic bacteria turn into gas and toxin-producing machines when they get access to FODMAPs. Within minutes, gut bacteria produce large amounts of methane, hydrogen, sulphur dioxide and hydrogen sulfide in the bowel. The more FODMAPs there are, the more acid and gas is produced. The increase in gas production stretches and distends the colon, overwhelming the intestine's ability to absorb the gases into the bloodstream where they can be excreted by the lungs. This is what causes the bloating, wind, abdominal pain, constipation and/or diarrhoea of IBS.[126]

The small size of FODMAPs means they move quickly through the gastrointestinal tract. Rapid movement of carbohydrates through the gut drags water with it and this increases the water content of the bowel and causes loose stools.[127]

A mild degree of malabsorption of FODMAPs is quite normal. Some FODMAPs are malabsorbed a little bit in all of us, and one in three healthy people will malabsorb some FODMAPs without any symptoms.

But why can some people eat FODMAP-rich foods and not get symptoms? Differences in the number and type of bacteria in the gut, and the level of sensitivity the gut has to distension, determine whether an individual will react to

---

[126] Barrett JS & Gibson PR, 2007, 'Clinical ramifications of malabsorption of fructose and other short-chain carbohydrates,' *Practical Gastroenterology*, vol. 53, pp. 51v65.

[127] Barrett JS et al, 2010, 'Dietary poorly absorbed, short-chain carbohydrates increase delivery of water and fermentable substrates to the proximal colon', *Alimentary Pharmacology and Therapeutics*, vol. 31, no. 8, pp. 874o182.

FODMAPs. The distension caused by ingestion of FODMAPs goes unnoticed by healthy people with a probiotic gut microbiome, but causes major symptoms in those with IBS and a dysbiotic gut microbiome.[128]

Everyone experiences some discomfort after a very high load of FODMAPs. Think about how you feel after a meal that includes large helping of legumes, beans, rice, lentils or chickpeas.

Baked beans are a very good start
Baked beans make you fart
The more you fart, the better you feel
It's baked beans for every meal.

Think about your own experiences with food. Maybe you are lactose intolerant and have noticed you can tolerate a cup of milk (full of lactose). Perhaps you always have digestive discomfort when you eat garlic or onions (which are full of fructans). If this is happening, then you are likely to be malabsorbing FODMAPs. Every time you eat foods with a high FODMAP content, you are feeding dysbiotic bacteria.

In the first phase of repairing your gut microbiome we are going to restrict FODMAPs so we can starve out dysbiotic bacteria. In the later stages of the program, they can be brought back into your diet. FODMAPs are safe to consume if you have a healthy microbiome and they don't give you gut symptoms.

---

[128] Goldstein R et al, 2000, 'Carbohydrate malabsorption and the effect of dietary restriction on symptoms of irritable bowel syndrome and functional bowel complaints', *Israel Medical Association Journal*, vol. 2, no. 8, pp. 583 587.

# Chapter 42

## The problem with genetically modified food

Genetically modified organisms (GMOs), most often foods like soy, corn, cotton, canola, sugar beets and alfalfa, have had a gene artificially inserted into them that allows them to resist *Roundup*, the most toxic pesticide on the planet. The deadly poisons carried by *Roundup* are glyphosate, which is a broad-spectrum herbicide, and polyethoxylated tallowamine (POEA). POEA is derived from animal fat. It helps the glyphosate penetrate the surface of plants and kill them.

A crop that is ready to be harvested can be sprayed with *Roundup*, which literally wipes out or damages every known weed, plant, bacteria, fungi, actinomycetes and yeasts, worm, beetle, insect, creepy crawly and tadpole, leaving a pristine, sterilised crop. *Roundup* persists in the soil for six months. According to the Environment Protection Authority about 45,000 tonnes of it is applied to American farms and lawns.

Researchers at France's University of Caen have shown that POEA is even more deadly to human embryonic, placental and umbilical cord cells than glyphosate itself.[129] This is a disturbing discovery indeed. However, this study was refuted by the makers of *Roundup* and the paper was subsequently retracted. The jury is out on the findings of this study.

Another study showed that glyphosate may induce cancer of the lymphatic system and is considered a risk factor for non-Hodgkin lymphoma (NHL).[130]

The problem for us is that the glyphosate and POEA penetrate directly into the crops, so when we eat GMO foods we are also swallowing these poisons. A disturbing study tested for glyphosate in the breastmilk of American women, and found high levels in 30% of the samples tested. Breastmilk glyphosate levels were found to be 760 to 1600 times higher than the European Drinking Water Directive allows for individual pesticides. This is strong evidence that glyphosate levels build up in our bodies over time.[131]

The poisons in *Roundup* also have an antibiotic-like effect on some probiotic gut bacteria and need to be avoided by anyone who is trying to restore a healthy microbiome. Unfortunately, the environmental authorities in most countries

---

[129] Seralini G et al. Long-term toxicity of a *Roundup* herbicide and a *Roundup*-tolerant genetically modified maize. Food and Chemical Toxicology. 2012:50(11); 4221-31

[130] Eriksson M et al, 2008, 'Pesticide exposure as risk factor for non-Hodgkin lymphoma including histopathological subgroup analysis', *International Journal of Cancer*, vol. 123, no. 7, pp. 1657l 063.

[131] Honeycutt Z & Rowlands H, 2014, 'Glyphosate testing full report: findings in American mothers' breast milk, urine and water', *Moms Across America*,
<www.momsacrossamerica.com/glyphosate_testing_results>, viewed 28 June 2017.

consider glyphosate to have low toxicity when used at the recommended doses. It appears *Roundup* is here to stay.

Another form of genetic modification of crops is to insert a gene that makes a deadly chemical called Bt toxin. Insects and bugs that feed on these crops get a dose of Bt toxin, which damages the insect's gut so severely that it causes massive uncontrolled leaky gut. Gut bacteria pour into the insect's bloodstream and kill it.

When we eat these crops, we also get a dose of Bt toxin. One study took the Bt toxin from a genetically modified corn plant and applied it to human gut cells. They found that Bt toxin also damages human cells and causes leakage by disrupting the barrier function.[132]

Even more disturbing is a study that found that Bt toxin was in the blood of 93% of pregnant women and about two-thirds of non-pregnant women. Bt toxin was also found in the cord blood of the pregnant women, which means it was also getting into their unborn babies.[133]

The bottom line is that the GMO crops on offer today kill probiotic gut bacteria and cause leaky gut. This is the exact opposite of what we are trying to do to restore a healthy gut environment and human health.

---

[132] Mesnage R et al, 2012, 'Cytotoxicity on human cells of Cry1Ab and Cry1Ac Bt insecticidal toxins alone or with a glyphosate-based herbicide', *Journal of Applied Toxicology*, vol. 33, no. 7, pp. 695-699.

[133] Aris A & Leblanc S, 2011, 'Maternal and fetal exposure to pesticides associated to genetically modified foods in eastern townships of Quebec, Canada', *Reproductive Toxicology*, vol. 31, no. 4, pp. 528ve33.

# Chapter 43

## The problem with food additives

Labels on manufactured food don't tell the whole truth. In Australia, food labelling tells you how much salt, sugar, carbohydrate, protein and fat solids are in the food but the nasty chemical food additives often fail to appear on the label. Some of the worst additives are found in packet chips, rice crackers, cheese crackers, two-minute noodles, luncheon meats, cordial drinks, chocolate-flavoured milk, frankfurts and sausages. Soft drinks, fruit juices and juice drinks are common offenders too, as they are full of artificial colours and packed with added refined sugars.

Australian food labelling laws allow manufacturers to get away with not listing any of the chemical additives in their product that make up 5% or less of the total product. This rule applies no matter how toxic or carcinogenic the chemical might be to people including pregnant and breast-feeding women, babies and children. Note that products with the label 'no artificial preservatives' does not mean that the product is preservative-free, and 'natural colour' doesn't mean that the product is free of chemically altered natural ingredients to give colour to processed foods that would otherwise look ugly. Any preservative works by killing bacteria, because bacteria cause food to spoil and reduces its shelf life.

Even if the labelling states that there are no added artificial flavouring or colouring agents used, this information can be very misleading. For example, a packet of a popular cheese-flavoured snacks that contains MSG (621), disodium guanylate (627) and disodium inosinate (631), which are linked to asthma, sleep disturbances, behavioural and learning problems in children, has an attention-grabbing label stating:

- No artificial colours
- No preservatives
- No artificial flavours.

The introduction of chemicals like these into the food chain has been linked to increases in disease rates. The damage they do to the gut microbiota is thought to be one of the key initiators of disease. For example, Australia now has one of highest asthma rates in the world at 14%. One in five Australian adolescents are estimated to have significant mental health problems, and teen suicide rates in males have quadrupled since the 1960s. At the rate the obesity epidemic is going, it is predicted that by 2025 every second child will be obese, not overweight, but largely obese! Heart disease is now the biggest killer in Western countries and, by the time they reach the age of 15 years, many of our children will have early heart disease.[134] The incidence of food allergies in kids is skyrocketing, as are autoimmune diseases in adults.[135]

Pressure from food manufacturers has meant that regulating authorities have not been keeping up with safeguarding our health for some time. Many food additives previously declared safe have been recalled and banned, but it is too late. The chemicals have already accumulated in our bodies and the damage has been done.

Chemical companies have discredited research by claiming that adverse effects in animal studies do not translate to people. But alarming results from one study showed that, when four common additives were eaten together, the damage from each additive was significantly greater. It was also demonstrated that the excessive and unnecessary amount of additives in a typical child's snack, such as chocolate milk and rice crackers or cordial and chips, stopped nerve cells growing and interfered with proper nerve-signalling systems.

There are now over 3200 chemicals registered as safe for use in food, despite the fact that there is little to no research into the safety, toxicity or cumulative health effects of these chemicals in people. Research conducted by Mount Sinai School of Medicine in New York found an average of 91 'industrial compounds, pollutants and chemicals' in the blood and urine of nine healthy volunteers and a total of 167 chemicals in the group. More frightening was the discovery that, of these chemicals, 76 cause cancer in humans or animals, 94 are toxic to the brain or nervous system, and 79 cause birth defects or abnormal development. None of the people tested worked with chemicals or lived near an industrial facility.

When trying to nurture healthy bacteria in the gut, it is vital to eliminate environmental toxins that damage the delicate balance of good bacteria. Seek out organic meats, fruit and vegetables wherever possible and avoid manufactured food.

[134]  Bridger T. Childhood obesity and cardiovascular disease. Paediatric Child Health 2009; 14(3);177-82.

[135]  Bach J et al. The effect of infections on susceptibility to autoimmune and allergic diseases. NEJM 2002; 347: 12: pp. 911-920.

# Chapter 44

# Getting rid of bad gut bacteria

So let's get to it. We start by doing what all healthy gut diet books fail to do. The critical first step in restoring global gut health is to eradicate the overgrowth of dysbiotic bacteria in the gut. Just as scientists always begin a scientific study with a germ-free animal, we are going to begin by creating a dysbiosis-free human. Without this step, other therapies are unlikely to have any lasting benefit.

So far we have repeatedly established that the presence of bad gut bacteria (dysbiosis) is the fundamental cause of the group of functional gut disorders we call chronic irritable bowel syndrome. Interestingly, the same gut dysbiotic pattern has been established in a host of other conditions such as autoimmune disease, CFS, IBD, RA, MS and many more. Many IBS sufferers also complain of milder cognitive symptoms as part of their problem and all patients with mental health conditions complain of IBS symptoms. There is an inextricable link between the integrity of the gut microbiome and normal brain function. It's called the gut-brain axis. There is no question that the clearing of toxic gut bacteria has to be a priority for restoring both good gut function and your sanity!

One of the ways that dysbiotic gut bacteria resist the natural defences of our gut that attempts to remove them is by forming a biofilm. Many bacteria that reside in the mucosal surfaces of the body secrete a protein and sugar mixture around themselves that acts like a slimy protective shell.

When dysbiosis occurs in the gut, the biofilm changes for the worse. A dysbiotic gut biofilm promotes gut inflammation and reduces absorption of nutrients and vitamins. This biofilm is designed to be tough. It is secreted to protect toxic bacteria, parasites and yeasts from the innate immune system of the gut and helps resist antibiotics. One such bug is *Pseudomonas*. Its biofilm is so tough that once it has attached itself to a bladder catheter or a central venous line it cannot be cleared by antibiotics. The only treatment is to remove the line. It's not the kind of biofilm we want in the gut.[136]

In a healthy gut that is filled with beneficial microflora, the biofilm they create are really just thin mucus layers that form part of the gut's natural outer mucous layer. This healthy film of intestinal and bacterial mucus allows the passage of food molecules and nutrients through the mucous layer to the cells lining the intestinal wall. A healthy probiotic gut biofilm is protective and anti-inflammatory, which is important when our guts are so prone to dysbiosis and leaky gut from food chemicals, pathogens and antibiotics.

---

[136] Macfarlane S & Dillon JF, 2007, 'Microbial biofilms in the human gastrointestinal tract', *Journal of Applied Microbiology*, vol. 102, no. 5, pp. 1187-1196.

Why do we begin by cleaning out bad bacteria? Because trying to reload your gut bacteria without first spring cleaning your gut of dysbiosis is like throwing a handful of grass seed into a paddock full of weeds and expecting to grow a lawn. It's not going to happen.

This is partly why probiotic supplements have been universally disappointing in human studies, despite showing amazing results in animals. The key difference is that mouse studies begin with a germ-free mouse. This is done either by genetic manipulation, by raising the mouse in a sterile environment or by eradicating the mouse gut microbiome with antibiotics. In a germ-free animal there is no resident gut bacteria waiting to kill off the new probiotics but this critical step is never followed in human probiotic studies.

The colon is such a rich and nourishing place to live that bacteria fight each other vigorously for their patch. Dropping a probiotic capsule into what is effectively two kilograms of hostile resident gut bacteria in the human colon is hardly a fair fight. While we can't render a human colon completely germ-free, using an antibacterial cleanse to lower the overgrowth of bad bacteria in your gut will make the microbiome reload much more effective. We can accelerate the process of repairing an unbalanced gut microbiome by weeding out the bad bacteria and making space for the good probiotic bacteria to repopulate the gut and create the new healthy microbiome.

Dysbiotic gut bugs do not give up easily. They compete incredibly hard for their patch of gut, producing their own antimicrobial substances and encasing themselves in their biofilms to protect them against invaders. They thrive in a lifestyle that is laden with chemicals, high in sugars, high in processed grains and low in fibrous vegetables. Toxic by-products of bad gut bacteria accumulate in the gut and damage both the healthy bacteria and the cells lining the gut. This results in a leaky gut and a continuous flood of toxic metabolites across the gut wall and into the bloodstream.

This process is associated with such a vast array of health problems that a cleanse and detoxification step has become the cornerstone of a successful microbiome restoration program. Eating prebiotic foods and taking probiotic bacteria alone is not enough.

# Chapter 45

# Phase One: Cleansing

This is not a detox. Although the idea of detoxing is very popular, nobody really knows exactly what detoxification diets actually are or what specific compounds or so-called toxins they are targeting for removal. There are a bevy of wildly different detoxification diets that range from just eating lemons through to wholesale laxative purges and everything in-between. The world of detoxification diets is a minefield and there is no research to prove their effectiveness. Stay well away from it.

Real detoxification – breakdown and deactivation of the multitude of chemicals, acids, aldehydes, pesticides, microbial toxins and other dangerous compounds that we consume each and every day – is done by our own good gut microbiome. At least half of detoxification is done this way, with the remainder being taken on by the liver. If you want a continuous, organic, natural detox, look no further than building yourself a healthy gut microbial zoo. This is exactly what this program is all about.

Phase One is like a bacterial sluicing of your bad gut microbes. This is a two-week dysbiosis cleansing program that is essentially a microbial clean-out of your gut. It is the essential first step to restoring a healthy gut microbiome.

## Cleanse bowels

This is the natural and gentle laxative-assisted removal of the faecal debris that is stuck in your colon. This debris is usually tenacious bits of old stool and it is especially common in people who have diverticulosis (abnormal pouches in the bowel) or slow colon transit constipation. It can also take the form of sticky, stringlike stool aggregates.

Bowel prep before a colonoscopy is an aggressive purge that is designed to empty the colon of its entire load of faecal matter in just a few hours by inducing explosive purging, but even this fails to clean out the cemented-on faeces in many people. I've seen many different kinds of poo aggregations during colonoscopies. They are smothered in dysbiotic bacteria and biofilms, which feed and house them and make them extremely difficult to clear from the bowel.

This is not how we are going to cleanse your bowels in this stage. By doing it more gently over a longer period, it will still be effective but will not risk dehydration or lose vital electrolytes and vitamins from your gut.

You will take just enough natural laxative to ensure your bowel moves daily. This will flush away the toxic bacterial load and begin to dislodge some bacterial biofilms from the large bowel. Trust me, I know full well that everybody has a different bowel transit time. I recommend you trial and adjust the type and amount of laxative needed until you get the correct dosage for your bowels. No stool or hard stool means you have used too little laxative and more than two stools a day or diarrhoea means you have used too much. Your aim is to find the dose that gives you a soft but formed bowel action every day that leaves you feeling satisfied and clean.

Every night during your dysbiotic cleanse, drink 100-200 ml of aloe vera juice mixed with 1-2 teaspoons of psyllium husk just before bed. Follow this with one glass of filtered water.

You can substitute the aloe vera juice with 50-100 ml of prune juice mixed with psyllium husk, or use aloe vera juice or prune juice by itself, or even a combination of aloe vera and prune juice mixed together if you have a very sluggish bowel habit. It has to suit your own bowel, so find the balance that works for you. If you cannot tolerate either of these natural laxatives, use what works for you.

Be aware that prune juice is high in sorbitol. Sorbitol is a FODMAP and it works as a laxative because it is not well absorbed by the gastrointestinal tract. If you have IBS and are sensitive to sorbitol, you may find the prune juice gives you bad bloating, wind, cramps and diarrhoea. If this happens, stop the prune juice and work with the other alternatives.

If you have IBS-C, the mixture described above may not be enough. In this case, add 12 teaspoons of a preparation that contains a mixture of magnesium oxide and magnesium carbonate to a glass of filtered water and drink that at night instead. Remember to start with a low dose and adjust it to suit your bowel.

If you have IBS-D, you may not need to do this step at all because it may aggravate your diarrhoea. You can still try taking psyllium husk in water at night to give your bowel motions some bulk without constipating you.

## Remove dysbiotic biofilm

Taking this extra step to remove the biofilm that protects dysbiotic bacteria in the gut will reduce the competitive environment in the gut and allow healthy probiotic gut bacteria to grow.

Each morning, take two teaspoons of apple cider vinegar mixed in a small glass of filtered water. Apple cider vinegar does not contain fructose, so it is safe to consume even if you are fructose-intolerant. The acetic acid component of vinegar gently cleanses away important minerals from the dysbiotic biofilm matrix.

Each morning, also take a complete digestive enzyme supplement on an empty stomach. Make sure it has a blend of lipase, protease and cellulase. If you take these enzymes with food, they will be consumed digesting food rather than working to disrupt biofilms. You can get these supplements from doctors, naturopaths and health food stores. In vitro studies have shown that the enzyme cellulase breaks down specific components of bacterial biofilms.[137] Adding the other enzymes will assist in degrading any lipid or protein component of the biofilm.

## Kill dysbiotic gut bacteria

This is the most important component of this phase. We don't want to wipe out any good bacteria that might be here, and that is why we are going to stay away from antibiotics. They have much too broad a kill range. They will take out both good and bad bacteria, leaving you open to yeast overgrowth or worse. To kill off bad microbes from the gut naturally, I advise taking a herbal antimicrobial blend. These formulas are specifically designed to manage dysbiosis and rid the small intestine and large bowel of dysbiotic bacteria, yeasts, fungi, intestinal worms and parasites. They contain extracts of herbs that have traditionally been used for their bitter, antimicrobial, antifungal, antiparasitic and antihelminthic actions. There are many such preparations and they are widely available. Find one from your local pharmacy, health food store, naturopath or doctor that contains any blend of the herbal extracts mentioned below.

Unlike antibiotics, herbal extracts also reduce gastrointestinal inflammation and do not alter gut permeability. They may also improve gut blood flow as well as reduce gut pain and bowel cramping. They kill microbes by blocking the construction of the vital bacterial cell walls.[138]

Oregano and thyme oils or extracts are the key ingredients. They are natural antiseptics that are active against many dysbiotic bacterial species that create dysbiosis in the gut. Traditionally, oregano and thyme oil have also been used for digestive complaints including nausea, poor digestion, wind, gas and bloating. You can take them on their own or in a commercial blend where they are usually mixed with other extracts such as lavender, wormwood, ginger, cinnamon, barberry, phellodendron or garlic. Any combination of these natural oils has an effective antiseptic effect on dysbiotic gut bacteria.

Begin with a low dose and increase by as much as you can tolerate. With a herbal blend start with one capsule daily, then increase to one capsule twice daily. If tolerated, increase to two capsules twice daily.

Some people may experience side effects such as stomach cramps, pains, agitation, diarrhoea or nausea. If you have any of these symptoms, stop taking it until the side effects disappear then start again at half the dose you were taking previously. If you develop a swollen tongue or throat, a rash or asthma, stop taking the herbal preparation immediately. This is an allergic response. You must see your doctor immediately and you cannot take this preparation again. People

---

[137] Loselle M et al. The use of cellulase in inhibiting biofilm formation from organisms commonly found on medical implants. Biofouling 2003; 19(2);77-85.

[138] Burt et al. Essential oils: There antibacterial properties and potential Int J Food Microbiol. 2004; 94(3); 223-253.

who are allergic to plants from the *Lamiaceae* family (mint, lavender, sage, and basil) should avoid oregano oil.

While the internet is rife with recipes for do-it-yourself thyme and oregano oil, I recommend purchasing a commercial product from a reputable pharmacy, drug store or health food shop as they are subject to regulations about preparation and safety. People also often get better results when they take it in a capsule form that is enteric coated to protect against degradation in the stomach.

Oregano and thyme oil is NOT advisable for infants and children. Pregnant or nursing women are also discouraged from using oregano and thyme oil. Oregano oil also has the potential to induce menstruation, and may be dangerous to an unborn child.

## Summary

| Step | Supplement | Dose | am | pm |
|---|---|---|---|---|
| Cleanse bowels | Aloe vera juice | 100-200 ml | | + |
| | Prune juice | 50-100 ml | | + |
| | Psyllium husk | 1-2 tsp | | + |
| Remove dysbiotic biofilm | Digestive enzyme | 1 capsule | + | |
| | Digestive enzyme | 1 capsule | | |
| Kill dysbiotic gut bacteria | Herbal antimicrobial | 2 tablets | + | + |

# Chapter 46

# Phase One: Low FODMAP diet

During Phase One of the program you will be eating low FODMAP food. By removing FODMAP sugars from your diet you will effectively starve bad bacteria right out of your gut. In addition, many IBS symptoms such as pain, bloating, wind, distension, constipation, diarrhoea and flatulence will be reduced.[139]

A low FODMAP diet is not for life. We will reintroduce some of these FODMAP foods again to nurture the good bacteria we will be reloading into your gut in Phase Two. So you only have to be strict with your food for the next two weeks.

Start by completely eliminating processed and chemical-laden foods from your diet. This means avoiding fast food and takeaways. Eat at home for the next seven to fourteen days so you can connect with and control your food. Start shopping more naturally from organic markets and biodynamic fresh food stores. This is your sample meal plan. It is designed to be clean, basic and FODMAP free. Recipes can be found at the end of this book.

## Low FODMAP meal plan

| Breakfast | Lunch | Dinner |
|---|---|---|
| Super green cleansing smoothie | Cleansing chicken salad | Cleansing fish Steamed vegetables |
| Cleansing quinoa fruit salad | Cleansing tuna salad | Cleansing meat Steamed vegetables |
| With each meal, drink 250 ml clean filtered water with fresh lemon slices | | |

If you are the sort of person who cannot survive on three meals a day, you have two choices. You can increase the size of each meal so you feel full enough to last to your next meal without snacking or you can snack between meals. My snack recommendations are a handful of walnuts and almonds with a sugar-free protein shake, or a banana with a sugar-free protein shake. You choose if and when you need it. If you are overweight, try and avoid snacking between meals.

---

[139] Ong DK et al, 2010, 'Manipulation of dietary short-chain carbohydrates alters the pattern of gas production and genesis of symptoms in irritable bowel syndrome', *Journal of Gastroenterology and Hepatology*, vol. 25, no. 8, pp. 1366of 73.

# FODMAP free foods

The meals suggested here are all low FODMAP and the foods listed below are a basic guide. I also highly recommend the Monash University Low FODMAP Diet app that is available on iTunes. It is by far the most up-to-date and comprehensive authority on FODMAP foods.

| Fruits | Vegetables | Other |
|---|---|---|
| Rockmelon, strawberry, raspberry, pineapple, blueberry, boysenberry, cantaloupe, banana, grapefruit, grape, paw paw, honeydew melon, kiwifruit, lemon, passionfruit, lime, mandarin, orange. | Yam, sweet potato, pumpkin, bamboo shoots, bean shoots, silverbeet, spinach, spring onion (green only), turnip, zucchini, squash, swede, tomato, beans (green), bok choy, broccoli, carrot, celery, capsicum, chives, corn, cucumber, eggplant, ginger, lettuce, parsnip, oregano, thyme, rosemary, chilli. | Yoghurt, hard cheeses, quinoa, buckwheat, rice, chia seed, sunflower seeds, almond meal, psyllium, oat bran, rice bran, peanuts, walnuts, pistachio nuts, almonds, most seeds, maple syrup, almond milk, coconut milk, LSA. |

# Alcohol

Alcohol is the most commonly abused drug on the planet, and some people struggle with my recommendation to stop drinking alcohol during this program. If it is impossible or very difficult for you to abstain from alcohol, make moderation your mantra. Beer, wine and spirits are FODMAP free.

If you must drink, you can consume a maximum of two glasses of beer or wine three times a week. Four alcohol-free days a week are very important. The phytonutrients contained in the grapes used to make wine may even be helpful to your gut microbiome. This level of alcohol consumption will not damage your gut microbiome or gut permeability.

However, I don't like spirits. The alcohol content of spirits is so high that it turns them into antiseptics that can kill gut bacteria, especially in the small bowel. The alcohol content can be reduced by diluting them, but mixers like Coke, tonic, lemonade and ginger ale are usually packed with sugar and do nothing but encourage dysbiosis.

## Water

One of the easiest ways to cleanse your system is to drink lots of non-chlorinated water. Ideally the water should be as pure as possible, so buy a bottle or get a filter fitted to your tap at home. Your body is 70% water by weight and we lose one litre a day through sweat, breathing and urination, so you need to drink to replenish your stores.

The Mayo Clinic recommends at least two litres of water per day, and more if it is hot or you are exercising. A good rule of thumb is that if your urine is pale and straw-coloured, you are well hydrated. If it is dark yellow, you need to drink more. Staying well hydrated allows your kidneys to remove water-soluble wastes more easily.

You can add a little lemon, or some nice organic herbal tea or just drink it straight. Water in alcohol doesn't count, but tea and coffee are fine in this stage. Tea is packed with brilliant antioxidants and coffee is bursting with chlorogenic acid and caffeine that stimulates some of the important detoxification pathways of the liver.

## Exercise

Exercising and staying fit improves gut microbial biodiversity. Studies of the gut bacteria of elite rugby players showed that they had more gut microbes, and a much wider variety of good microbes, than men who did not exercise. The athletes also had lower levels of inflammation and faster metabolism of sugars. The higher protein component of the athletes' diet also correlated with healthier gut bacteria. The research is clear: exercising encourages a rich and healthy gut microbiome and a good protein intake helps too.

It is an excellent idea to start your fitness regime in the cleansing phase so that it is established when we move to reloading your gut with good bacteria. Aim for 30 to 40 minutes of moderate intensity aerobic exercise (brisk walking, cycling, aerobics or swimming) three to four times a week, plus one or two sessions of strengthening exercises (weight training, yoga or pilates).

Try to do some form of exercise every day, and preferably at the same time every day. You only need to do 20 minutes, but it needs to have a high-intensity component. Studies have also shown that the most efficient way to promote bowel function, proper bowel evacuation and burn fat every time you work out is to do High Intensity Interval Training. Simply put, this means varying the pace by doing sets of 30 seconds of fast activity and 45 seconds of slow activity, as well as varying the type of exercise.

The HIIT program only requires you to commit to 30 minutes of exercise a day. You can start with 10 minutes a day, then extend this by one minute each time you work out until you are fit enough to do the full 30 minutes. If at first you can't sprint, just go as fast as you can for each high-intensity cycle. Try to do a different type of cardio each time to maximise the benefit.

# Meditation

Almost all of my patients report that their stress levels influence not only their mood and wellbeing but their gut symptoms as well. The chronic elevation of stress hormones is damaging to your gut microbiome. Try to find the positives in the challenges that life throws at you as well as the negatives. Balancing your emotional response to stress will make you more optimistic and focused on your health.

Regardless of whether you have a major stress in your life or lots of smaller stresses, practicing a relaxation technique like yoga, tai chi, meditation or prayer may be helpful. There are numerous health benefits of meditation but the calming effects on your mind and the lowering of stress hormones are especially helpful to your gut microbiome. They lead to a reduction in a very important neurotransmitter hormone call corticotrophin release factor (CRF). CRF is secreted by the hypothalamus and mediates the adrenal hormones that are involved in the 'fight or flight' stress response. Having too much CRF leads to a whole-body stress response that can cause unwanted changes in the gut microbiota. Practising yoga and meditation for just 10 minutes a day will lead to benefits.

To meditate, find a quiet time of the day when you won't be disturbed. Sit comfortably in a chair or cross-legged on a cushion on the floor. Close your eyes, and focus on your breathing. Take four counts to inhale, pause, then take four counts to exhale.

Continue this breathing pattern and relax your body. Start with your feet and work all the way up to the crown of your head. Next, focus your relaxation on your eyes and the muscles of your face and then move to feel the relaxation deep in the temples at the side of the head.

Once your whole body and face are relaxed, start to clear your mind of all thoughts. Concentrate on stillness. Gradually let your mind become calm. Settle into a nurturing feeling of complete warmth and calmness. Feel the peace permeate your mind until you are bathed in complete stillness.

Practice this for as long as it takes you to reach a feeling of peace in your body and mind. Mediate every day to obtain maximum effect.

# What to expect

Despite what you might think, this bacterial wipe-out phase often leaves people feeling great. The minute you start dropping the dysbiotic bacteria count in your gut, bloating and distension reduce, energy increases, mood elevates and concentration becomes more focus and sustained.

Phase One is easy to implement, and you will probably feel much better in just a few days. You may need to make some modifications to the supplement regime or the diet to suit your own unique set of health circumstances or food sensitivities. That's OK. Do the best you can. Kickstart your microbiome repair and enjoy the surge in wellbeing.

# Chapter 47

# Phase Two: Two basic principles

You've just spent two weeks weeding your gut of biofilms, damaging bacteria and removing the toxic metabolic by-products that they make. The entire purpose of this gut eradication process was to create space to sow a new healthy probiotic garden in your gut. You only have a few days before undesirable bugs will begin migrating back, so it's essential to start this reloading phase as soon as you can.

The focus in this phase of the program moves from killing bad dysbiotic bugs to promoting the growth of healthy probiotic bugs and preventing a recurrence of gut dysbiosis, leaky gut and formation of unhealthy biofilms. Having cleansed away the toxin-producing bacteria that irritate the gut nervous system, you are now in a stronger position to add many of the foods that once irritated your gut back into your diet. But you must do it slowly.

It is important to start testing a broad range of foods, because they are necessary to feed good gut bacteria. This is why I don't recommend following the strict FODMAP-free diet for a prolonged period. You may experience some relief from your symptoms by removing FODMAPs from your diet, but you will never cure your condition this way. FODMAP foods are like fertiliser for your gut garden. You don't have to eat lots of them but your good microbes will thrive if you eat just a little of them.

Be gentle with your gut. Add these foods back one at a time and in small, measurable amounts. Everybody, even those with a healthy gut, can still have one or two trigger foods that simply do not and probably never will agree with them. A controlled eating plan will let you identify those foods that you may need to avoid completely.

There are two basic principles involved in reloading your gut microbiome. These are things that everyone should do to ensure they create and maintain a healthy gut.

## Principle one: Eat a natural diet made up of wholefoods

Eating this way might sound like a lot of work, especially if you are used to a diet of fast junk food. However, your life will change if you begin to take an interest in the stuff you put in your mouth to fuel your body. Remember, the food you eat is like the soil your body extracts its nutrients from, and your intestine puts down roots in this soil to do that extracting. You wouldn't plant your garden in a toxic junk soil, so why do that to your precious body? A simple change in mindset is all it takes.

To do this, you will probably have to become more interested in food and cooking. If you cut out all processed flours, sugars, fast foods and refined seed oils and replace them with vegetables, fruits, nuts, gluten-free grains and fish, you are off to a great start! Choose foods that are rich in plant-based carbohydrates and beneficial microbes. Fermented foods like sauerkraut, kefir, fermented coconut yoghurt, fermented vegetables, kimchee, cultured sauces and dips with sour cream and yoghurt and drinks like probiotic beverages are all great sources of healthy bacteria.

## Principle two: Supplement your diet with nutrients

There are a few key micronutrients like probiotics, glutamine, prebiotics and vitamins that your gut requires to maintain structural and functional integrity. They will help your gut lining, nervous system and immune system to stay healthy and continue the vital processes of constant repair, energy and renewal.

# Chapter 48

## Phase Two: Microbiome reload diet

Regrowing a healthy gut microbiome is all about the type of food that you feed it. Learning how to eat for your gut microbiome is the foundation of any program designed to restore the balance and biodiversity of gut bacteria and prevent health issues. It's one of the most important things you can do to lose weight, maintain healthy body fat, restore happiness, improve sleep, reduce anxiety, stop the pro-inflammation effects of dysbiotic bacteria, prevent heart disease and stop the immune overactivity that initiates autoimmune disease. Studies have shown that the right foods can also help heal the gut wall.

The microbiome reload diet is an ancestral diet, meaning it is a way of eating that takes us back to the days when we had to eat wholefoods that were either caught or grown in nature. It avoids modern processed foods and chemicals wherever possible. Although it looks a little bit like the Paleo or 'caveman' diet, it also contains some of the foods our more recent ancestors ate.

The first step is to change your mindset. You have to really commit, at a deep level within your subconscious, to follow a set of healthy eating principles that will govern your life from this point forward. Tell yourself that this is now your personal health philosophy. This change in mindset is simple. It is a commitment to eat only what Mother Earth provides. Eat what grows in the ground or on a tree or bush, swims in the ocean, or walks on and eats grass. Don't eat anything that comes out of a factory.

The good news is that studies show that you can make positive or negative changes to your gut microbiota within one day of changing your diet. This is how powerful the microbiome reload diet really is. If you stick to it, you will profoundly change the probiotic levels in your gut. But you do need to maintain it in the long term.

## Natural eating

To begin with, I recommend you follow the seven tenets of natural eating. This alone will stop the death of your gut microbiome and begin to restock the shelves of your intestines with good microbes.

| The seven tenets of natural eating |
| --- |
| No processed food |
| No gluten (wheat, rye, barley) |
| No GMO foods |
| No processed dairy (store-bought milk, cream, ice-cream) |
| No refined sugar/fructose (including artificial sweeteners) |
| No margarines/vegetable/seed oils |
| Go organic |

## Microbiome reload diet rules

Print these off and stick them on the fridge. You need to read them regularly to remind yourself about your new attitude to food. These rules are also incorporated into the meal plan that follows.

1. **Eliminate sugar**
   This includes fruit juices and sports drinks that contain high fructose corn syrup, table sugar. Do not add extra sugar to food and avoid food with added sugars.
2. **Eat healthy fats**
   Healthy fats include coconut oil, grass-fed butter, ghee, olive oil or MCT oil.
3. **Reduce gluten**
   This includes wheat, rye, barley based breads, cereals, and pastas. Do not make the mistake of resorting to gluten-free junk food, which can be full of potato starch, corn starch and soy.
4. **Remove all refined seed oils**
   These include grain-derived oils and all vegetable oils such as corn, sunflower, safflower, peanut, macadamia, soy and canola and unstable polyunsaturated oils like margarine and peanut oil.

5.  **Eat the right carbohydrates**
    These include brown rice, wild rice, quinoa, buckwheat, sweet potato, carrot, turnips and amaranth.

6.  **Eliminate all synthetic food chemical additives, preservatives, colourings, and flavourings**
    This includes aspartame, MSG, dyes, emulsifiers, food colourings, preservatives, antioxidants, antiquating agents, flavour enhancers, food acids and thickeners like corn starch and wheat starch.

7.  **Switch to grass-fed meats**
    Eat free-range eggs, chickens, turkeys and ducks. Eat significant amounts of pastured, grass-fed meat such as beef, lamb, buffalo, kangaroo and venison.

8.  **Eat fresh seafood**
    Include small red and white fish or baby fish and shellfish, but limit large fish like swordfish and tuna because of their high mercury content.

9.  **Soak your legumes**
    Nuts, beans, and lentils should be activated by soaking overnight in water to remove toxic phytates. Even then they should only be eaten in small amounts and perhaps not at all if you already have autoimmune disease.

10. **Remove all processed dairy**
    Dairy products from grass-fed animals can be consumed in small amounts. Most people can eat full-fat whole milk, butter, some hard cheeses and yoghurt from grass-fed cows.

11. **Switch to organic fruits and vegetables**
    Find a farmers' market, read the labels at the supermarket or order online from an organic grocer.

12. **Cook your food gently**
    Use a steamer or dry bake them in an oven. Do not use a microwave or deep fryer.

13. **Add fresh herbs and spices liberally**
    Use fresh leaves and grind high-quality, recently purchased seeds yourself, rather than powders.

14. **Eat fermented foods**
    These include kefir, yogurt, cheese, miso, kimchi, sauerkraut cabbage, tempeh, kombucha, pickles, pickled artichokes, eggplant and cucumbers. If you are new to fermented foods, start by adding them in very, very small quantities until you get used to them.

15. **Eat bone broth**
    Bone broths are nutrient-dense, easy to digest, rich in flavour and they boost gut healing. I recommend consuming one cup of broth twice daily. Many store-bought beef and chicken stocks are lacking in nutrients, so to get the benefits of real bone broth and real bone broth benefits, buy it from

an organic butcher or make it yourself at home. A simple recipe is included in the back of this book.

The overriding rule of the microbiome reload diet is 'feed your microbiome first and yourself second'. Practically, this means starting your main evening meal with a green salad and finishing with meat and vegetables. Think of the green salad as your gut microbial medicine but, instead of taking it as tablets, you take it as food. That's pretty cool.

This is also easy to do when you are eating out – just order your first course from the salad menu. Ask them to hold the dressing though, because restaurant-made dressings are full of sugar, emulsifiers, preservatives and seed oils. If you want your salad with dressing, ask for extra-virgin olive oil and freshly squeezed lemon juice or balsamic vinegar. All good restaurants will be very happy to oblige.

A leafy green salad provides fibre to give you a great bowel action every day but, more importantly, it powers up your microbiome. Leafy green vegetables like spinach, beetroot leaves, bok choy, endive, radicchio, rocket, cos, kale, red oak and other lettuce leaves are packed full of a newly discovered carbohydrate called sulfoquinovose. Sulfoquinovose is such a rich fuel for good gut microbes that eating it produces the same microbe-boosting effect on the gut as taking a probiotic. Research has confirmed the importance of eating your greens, and the greener the better. Dump that pale iceberg lettuce for the deepest darkest leaves you can find.

One of my friends has become such a convert to the benefits of the 'green leaves as medicine regime' that he not only keeps his own gut spinning over beautifully with this simple dietary routine, but he has also converted his entire pro-cycling team to this regime with fantastic results.

Another tip to help improve the first phase of digestion when you are starting a more rich and varied diet is to boost your stomach acid secretion at the start of your main meals. Many people suffer low stomach acid secretion and they can feel sick when they eat meat. Either put oil and vinegar on your salad or have a shot of two teaspoons of organic apple cider vinegar mixed in a cup of water at the start of the meal. This works beautifully. It's not rocket science. It's just basic stomach digestion physiology. If taking the vinegar upsets your stomach, you are already making enough stomach acid naturally and don't need the extra shot.

The fermented foods suggested can be bought from organic health food stores and farmers' markets or can be prepared at home. You can download a multitude of recipes for making fermented foods. If you are eating a fermented food for the first time, test a tiny amount until your gut gets used to it. Some people cannot tolerate fermented foods no matter how hard they try. If that is you, just eliminate them from the meal plan.

Finally, you will see that every second breakfast in the suggested meal plan is served with a cup of stewed apple. Remember, in this phase you are allowed to bring back FODMAP foods as long as you are not intolerant to them. Probiotics also love FODMAPs so it's fine to eat a little of them as long as you don't have dysbiosis.

Studies in humans and rats have shown that apple pectin increases the levels of very important probiotic gut bacteria. Apple pectin also significantly increases the expression of genes that code for the production of butyrate.[140] [141]Pectin slows glucose and cholesterol absorption, which may benefit people with diabetes and elevated cholesterol. Several studies have also shown that pectins have specific anti-cancer properties that allow them to bind to certain tumour cells and kill them. This has led to the development of several anti-cancer drugs that have been produced directly from pectin.[142]

If you have had problems with *Candida* overgrowth, you should get it treated and repopulate your bowel with a healthy microbiome. Stewed apple will help you to regrow a healthy gut microbiome that will defend you and block out *Candida*. If you are severely fructose intolerant you may have to eliminate the stewed apple, but give it a try. Start with one teaspoon and see if you can tolerate it. It doesn't matter if you have to leave it out of your diet. Some people are so sensitive to fructose that they can never eat apples or pears. Some improve drastically once they rebuild a strong gut microbiome.

## Ten-day microbiome reload meal plan

This meal plan is just a recommended eating schedule. Feel free to switch the meals around and change them to suit your palate and your lifestyle. Substitute alternatives for any meat, fruits or vegetables that you know you react to. The guiding principles of what your meals should look like and how to prepare food that will boost your gut bacteria and health are clear. Learn to apply these principles, and enjoy your food. Recipes are included in the back of this book.

|       | **Breakfast** | **Lunch** | **Dinner** |
|-------|---------------|-----------|------------|
| **Day 1** | • 1 serve stewed apple and cinnamon <br> • 2 tbs probiotic yoghurt or kefir <br> • ½ cup blueberries, | • Tuna and green salad | • Spinach and radicchio salad <br> • Pesto chicken and vegetables |

---

[140] Licht TR et al, 2010, 'Effects of apples and specific apple components on the cecal environment of conventional rats: role of apple pectin', *BMC Microbiology*, vol 10, no. 13, doi: 10.1186/1471-2180-10-13.

[141] Chung WS et al, 2016', Modulation of the human gut microbiota by dietary fibres occurs at the species level', *BMC Biology*, vol. 14, no. 3, doi: 10.1186/s12915-015-0224-3.

[142] Sathisha UV et al, 2007, 'Inhibition of galectin-3 mediated cellular interactions by pectic polysaccharides from dietary sources', *Glycoconjugate Journal*, vol. 24, no. 8, pp. 497r507.

|  |  |  |  |
|---|---|---|---|
|  | raspberries or strawberries<br>• 1 tsp LSA (ground linseed, sunflower, almonds) |  |  |
| **Day 2** | • Omelette with spinach and lemon kale | • Chicken soup with avocado salad | • Beetroot, rocket and cabbage salad<br>• Steak and winter vegetables |
| **Day 3** | • Grilled mushroom salad<br>• ½ cup stewed apple and cinnamon | • Vegetable stack | • Spinach and kale salad<br>• Chilli ginger prawns |
| **Day 4** | • Poached eggs on quinoa and vegetables | • Beef soup with baked sweet potato | • Spinach, celery and cabbage salad<br>• Fish and cauliflower rice |
| **Day 5** | • ½ cup ancestral muesli<br>• 1 cup stewed apple and cinnamon<br>• 2 tbs probiotic yoghurt<br>• 1 tbs fresh raspberries | • Salmon and rocket salad | • Spinach, kale and red oak salad<br>• Roast lamb and winter vegetables |
| **Day 6** | • Fruit salad with coconut | • Chicken soup with cucumber salad | • Cos, endive and kale salad<br>• Zucchini noodles with meatballs and Napoli sauce |
| **Day 7** | • Ancestral porridge<br>• 1/2 cup stewed apple and cinnamon | • Grilled chicken with rice and vegetables | • Spinach, rocket and pear salad<br>• Tamarind and lime salmon with steamed vegetables |

| Day 8 | • Green smoothie bowl | • Minestrone with fennel and orange salad | • Spinach and beetroot salad<br>• Chicken stir fry |
|---|---|---|---|
| Day 9 | • Green cacao shake<br>• 1/2 cup stewed apple and cinnamon | • Beef soup with mixed vegetables | • Spinach and butter lettuce salad<br>• Tuna with wasabi mash |
| Day 10 | • Almond banana smoothie | • Baked sweet potato salad | • Kale, parsley and parmesan salad<br>• Eggplant parmigiana |

# Chapter 49

# Phase Two: Lifestyle and supplements

In addition to the microbiome reload diet, some simple lifestyle changes are needed to rebuild your gut microbiome. They aren't complicated or arduous and they don't cost a lot of money. There are only a few extras that you need to help you along the way. Some are lifestyle changes and some are supplements, but they all boost the health and richness of your gut bacteria.

## Get outdoors

This is just as important for your microbiome as anything else we have discussed so far. Research shows that walking outdoors showers us in a microscopic veil of good bacteria, yeast and viruses. You can't help but inhale them, swallow them and get them all over your skin. All of this enriches your microbial community. It's even more exciting when you go to the beach. The oceans are teaming with beneficial microbes. They contain around half the total biomass of living microbes on the planet. It's estimated that almost 10 million viruses and a host of other bacteria and archaea are contained in every drop of seawater. Imagine how many bugs we get in our mouths, hair, skin, ears and gut from a humble trip to the seaside and a dip in the ocean.[143]

Humans have been a part of the great microbial life cycle for 2.5 million years. It's only since the discovery of penicillin and antiseptics that we began to move out of it. There is no doubt that our gut microbiome physically needs to be part of it. This prescription is simple. Go outside. Walk, sniff the air, touch the plants, dig your toes in the soil and swim in the ocean. Play with your dog. People who have a pet have significantly more biodiversity in their gut microbiomes than those who don't. In fact, you share microbes with all members of your family – human and animal.[144]

## Probiotic

Most of us are lacking in the important bugs from the genus *Bifidobacterium* and *Lactobacillus*. Let's be honest, apart from *E. coli*, *Streptococcus*, *Saccharomyces boulardii* and soil-based probiotics, all probiotics are mostly blends of various strains of *Bifidobacterium* and *Lactobacillus* anyway.

---

[143] Marathe P, 2013, 'A whole new world: scientists discover abundant viruses living under the sea', *Yale Scientific*, vol.14, no. 6, 20:38.

[144] Song et al, 2013, 'Cohabiting family members share microbiota with one another and with their dogs', *eLife*, doi: 10.7554/eLife.00458

While the medical literature is awash with studies proclaiming the benefits of different probiotic strains, they have not turned out to be the panacea that animal studies promised they were going to be. Any discussion about the specific benefits of one probiotic over another is still premature. It would take another book to discuss the volume of research that has been performed in this area.

That being said, probiotic capsules will help maintain the biodiversity of your gut microbiome. For thousands of years, we have eaten a multitude of probiotic bacteria that have been growing on food or passed onto food from our filthy unwashed hands. In these modern times of fastidious hygiene, we no longer get enough top-up probiotic bacteria from our fingers, food and animals. Taking a probiotic capsule can act as a daily boost of good bacteria. But the bacterial strains contained in probiotic capsules will only last in the gut for a couple of weeks. If you are going to supplement with them, you need to keep taking them intermittently for the long term.

The strains most frequently cited are *E. coli nissle*, *Lactobacillus rhamnosus*, *L. casei*, *L. plantarum*, *L. acidophilus*, *L. helveticus*, *L. reuteri*, *Bidifobacterium longum*, *B. infantis*, and *Saccharomyces boulardii*. I recommend a high-quality blend of different *Lactobacillus* and *Bifidobacterium* strains. The exceptions are for IBS-C, where *E. coli nissle* has been shown to be the most effective probiotic. For traveller's diarrhoea and IBS-D, *Saccharomyces boulardii* has been most effective and *L. helveticus* with *B. longum* is best for anxiety and mood disturbances. Crohn's and ulcerative colitis have generally responded in part to broad spectrum blends of multiple different strains.

Take the probiotic once or twice daily on an empty stomach. Ensure that there are at least 20 billion cfu per capsule. Keep them in the fridge – probiotic bacteria thrive at human body temperature, which is 36-37.5 °C. Once they are warmed up, probiotic bacteria will die unless they are inside your bowel where they get food.

Note that people who are prone to bacterial overgrowth of the small intestine may not tolerate oral probiotic capsules. They may aggravate the symptoms of SIBO by adding more bacteria to the already inappropriately high bacterial overgrowth.

## Glutamine

Glutamine is an amino acid derived from protein. It is a critical energy source that allows our gut lining to function properly. Around one-third of total glutamine usage by our bodies occurs in the intestinal epithelial cells. It's no surprise that glutamine depletion is associated with impaired intestinal structure and poor gut epithelial cell function. Glutamine is also necessary for normal function of the tight junctions of the intestines. Glutamine supplementation has been shown to reduce gut permeability and it also prevents the development of leaky gut that occurs with use of aspirin and other NSAIDs.

People who are critically ill or who have had major surgery often cannot eat food. They are fed intravenously with liquid nutrients supplied directly into their blood vessels through a tube. The nutrients bypass the gut completely, so the gut microbes and gut cells don't get adequate nutrition. This leads to gut lining damage and leaky gut and puts patients at risk of infection from gut bacteria leaking across the gut wall into blood. Adding glutamine to the intravenous feed helps maintain a healthy gut lining and reduces leaky gut. It has been used extensively this way to help repair gut permeability defects in critically ill people.[145]

When starting a glutamine supplement, start at two grams daily. You can add glutamine powder to a shake, mix it in water or add it to your fibre supplement. Increase your daily dose by two grams each week until you reach the optimum amount of eight grams a day. If you have Crohn's disease or colitis, increasing the glutamine to 16 grams a day, but take it in two doses – eight grams in the morning and eight at night – to avoid bloating or nausea.

## Prebiotic fibre

Many years ago, when I got sick of smoggy city life, I spent a week in a health retreat with 30 other disaffected city slickers. It was a picturesque resort, full of organic vegetarian food, located in the tropical hinterland of Queensland. I loved the idea of eating a high-fibre diet and loading up on organic fruit and vegetables and salads. It sounded like the perfect solution to restore my gut bacteria and health. Despite the positive effects of this diet, like boundless energy, clear skin, bright eyes and a sharper mind, I started to bloat. By day six I was so constipated and bloated that my belly was protruding out beyond the fit of any pants I had brought with me.

My gut was in shock. It couldn't tolerate the massive increase in fibre load that I was consuming. A boatload of laxatives later and the sluice gates opened. It was like popping a balloon with a pin and the bloating went down. The lesson is that not everyone can handle the broad range of different fibres fermenting in their gut when they significantly increase their fibre intake.

Plant foods contain a mix of three types of fibre. Soluble fibre is partially broken down by our gut bacteria to a gel-like material that adds moisture to the stool. This is great for keeping the bowels regular. It is found in oats, psyllium, nuts, bran, seeds, beans and fruit.

Insoluble fibre is the tough fibrous indigestible component of the plants like legumes, vegetable and fruit skins, barley, oats, carrots. It doesn't absorb moisture or dissolve in water. It is tough, isn't broken down much by our gut bacteria and forms the bulk of the stool. But it can lead to distension, hard bowel motions and constipation when eaten in large amounts.

---

[145] Hond ED et al, 1999, 'Effect of glutamine on the intestinal permeability changes induced by indomethacin in humans', *Alimentary Pharmacology and Therapeutics*, 1999, vol. 13, no. 5, pp. 6791685.

And then there is resistant starch. These are the starch components of foods that we can't break down and that pass undigested into the colon. Our colonic gut probiotic bacteria thrive on resistant starch. It is found in sweet potatoes, beans, nuts, oat, bananas and spinach. Most healthy foods like fruits, gluten-free grains, legumes and other vegetables contain a mix of these three types of fibre.

Even eating this microbiome reload diet, most of us will only manage to pack in around 40 grams of fibre each day. That's great, considering that the average dietary intake of people in the West is just 5 to 15 grams a day, and the recommended daily intake is between 20 and 25 grams a day. In some people, this increase in fibre may cause some bloating and constipation, while in others it may bring on diarrhoea. We know that people can handle much higher intakes that this – hunter-gatherer societies eat almost 10 times this amount of fibre. But people who are new to a high-fibre diet simply can't motor through the sheer volume of food that it requires to reach intakes of 50 to 60 grams of fibre per day. And if they did, they would have serious bloating issues. For most people, an intake of around 30 grams of fibre a day is enough to significantly change your microbiome. Don't despair if you can't tolerate all the salads, fruit and vegetables recommended in this diet. Take it slowly at first, then build.

Fibre supplements can be of enormous value in building a healthy gut microbial zoo. Taken once a day, they help to maintain a good regular bowel motion and take the pressure off your daily requirement to eat quite so much fibre. The best supplements are soluble fibre and resistant starch, because they are essentially just prebiotic foods. That means they help the probiotic bacteria to grow and form soft stools that are easy to pass.

We know that eating more fibre, by boosting your intake of fresh vegetables, fruit and unrefined whole grains, will reduce your risk of diabetes, obesity, Crohn's and colitis. Recent scientific research published in the journal *Cell Host & Microbe* has revealed just how dietary fibre improves the health of your bowel and reduces disease risk.

Mice fed a low-fibre diet developed defects in the protective gut mucous barrier, making it too leaky. This increased the risk of bad bacteria crossing the gut, which led to inflammation and disease. Remember, a healthy relationship with our gut bacteria relies on them being kept at a respectable distance from the cells lining your gut so as not to trigger our complex gut immune system. And, it is having a healthy gut barrier and not a 'leaky' one that does this.

Interestingly, this damage could be repaired in those mice by receiving a faecal transplant from healthy mice, which had been fed a high-fibre diet.[146]

However, supplementing with the probiotic bifidobacteria could not repair the damage. How does it do this? By altering the bacterial make-up of the gut microbiome, of course.

---

146  Schoeder B et al. Bifidobacteria or Fibre Protects against Diet-Induced Microbiota-Mediated Colonic
Mucus Deterioration. Cell Host & Microbe 2108, (in press) http://dx.doi.org/10.1016/j.chom.2017.11.004

Mice fed the low-fibre diet had an unhealthy or dysbiotic bowel microbiome. It took FMT from mice fed a high-fibre diet that allowed them to grow a probiotic microbiome to significantly change the levels of good bacteria again and allow the damaged gut barrier to heal.

A commonly available prebiotic product is inulin, a long chain fructose-based fibre from the chicory root. Be cautious with it, as it is a fructo-oligosaccharide and one study showed that it could cause flatulence and bloating in some people unless the level was maintained below 10 grams per day. Our probiotic gut microbiome thrives on inulin, so any addition of it is beneficial. Any resistant starch can also be added as a probiotic supplement.

It is much less stressful and less likely to cause bloating and gas if you eat as much natural, plant-based fibre-rich food that feels comfortable for your gut and take a prebiotic fibre supplement nightly. Start with two grams a day and see how well you tolerate it. Increase the dose by two grams a day until you reach eight grams. In general, stick to no more than 10 grams of fibre supplement a day. If you feel great on 10 grams a day but you want to increase the fibre supplement to give your microbiome a super boost, let your gut decide the dose. Some people need much more.

## Vitamin D

We are all familiar with the role that vitamin D plays in growing strong bones but it is a critical player in the gut too. Vitamin D strengthens tight junctions and helps make them resistant to damage from chemicals. It also promotes intestinal epithelial cell repair after injury to the gut lining.

Vitamin D deficiency is a major problem in Australia because of our fear of sun exposure and our high incidence of skin cancer. Supplement with 3000 iu of vitamin D daily and have regular checks to make sure the level of vitamin in your blood is at the high end of the normal range.

## Daily gut supplement regime

| Supplement | Dose | Time |
|---|---|---|
| Probiotic | 20-60 billion | Once daily |
| Glutamine | 6-8 g | Once daily |
| Prebiotic fibre | 6-10 g | Once daily |
| Vitamin D | 3000 iu | Once daily |

# Conclusion

We coexist with a robust community of gut microbes. The composition of that community is hugely important and is a delicate balance of our genetics, diet and lifestyle. The gut microbiome is now firmly established as a crucial element in human health and disease. The shift from a diet made up of wild, natural food to one of highly processed food has critically damaged our once robust and protective gut microbiome. Added to this, our misplaced fear of bacteria and overuse of antibiotics have seen us exchange death from infection for a life of decay at the hands of allergies, chronic inflammatory heart and brain conditions and a host of autoimmune diseases. The prevailing chronic diseases of this century may all be the result of these changes in our precious gut microbiome.

What I sincerely hope you have gained from this book is the insight to understand your gut bacteria, the confidence to trust your gut feelings about your health and the knowledge you need to begin the journey back to ultimate health by recreating the profoundly protective gut microbiome that nature and evolution has provided us with.

Go forth with this knowledge, forever be a student and heal yourself from within.

# Recipes: Low FODMAP diet

## Breakfast recipes

*Super green cleansing smoothie*

### Ingredients
- ½ cup baby spinach leaves
- ½ cup kale, chopped
- ¼ cup frozen blueberries, strawberries, raspberries or banana
- 1 teaspoon powdered spirulina or chlorella or both
- ½ cup ice (from filtered water)
- 1 cup almond milk, coconut milk, coconut water or rice milk

### Method
Place the ingredients in a blender and blend until smooth and frothy.

### Benefits
This smoothie is packed with phytonutrients and antioxidants that will not only help fight off dysbiotic bacteria but will help with waste removal and provide prebiotic support to encourage regrowth of good probiotic bacteria in the gut. The boost of spirulina and chlorella assists in removal of heavy metals, has anti-microbial effects against *Candida*, promotes the growth of good probiotic bacteria, boosts gut immune defences, lowers blood pressure and cholesterol, prevents atherosclerosis in the brain and heart, boosts energy and may help with weight loss.

*Cleansing quinoa fruit salad*

This can be eaten for breakfast on alternate days to the green shake.

### Ingredients
- Any three of these fresh organic fruits
  - Strawberries
  - Pawpaw
  - Kiwifruit
  - Rockmelon
  - Honeydew melon
  - Grapes
  - Pineapple
  - Blueberries
  - Banana
- 2 tablespoons cooked quinoa
- Pulp of 1 passionfruit (optional)
- 1 tablespoon pepitas
- 2 tablespoons natural probiotic yoghurt

### Method
Toss the fruits in a bowl. Mix through the quinoa and passionfruit (if using). Top with pepitas and yoghurt.

### Benefits
These are low-GI fruits, so they will not cause a rapid rise in blood sugar nor will they supply any sugars to dysbiotic gut bacteria. The yoghurt supplies some probiotic bacteria to fight dysbiotic bacteria and the quinoa gives some gluten-free complex carbohydrates for energy and nourishes your good gut bacteria.

# Lunch recipes

*Cleansing chicken salad*

You can pack this into a glass container and take it with you to work. If any of these foods upset your gut, just leave them out for the time being.

***Ingredients (serves 2)***
- 300 gm grilled chilli-rubbed organic free-range chicken or turkey breast
- ½ cup sliced celery
- ½ cup sliced red capsicum
- ½ cup fresh cucumber
- ½ cup butter lettuce and red oak lettuce
- 2 tablespoons cooked brown rice
- 8 cherry tomatoes (halved)
- 1 tablespoon chopped almonds

***Dressing***
- Lemon juice or apple cider vinegar
- Cold-pressed extra virgin olive oil
- Pepper
- Chopped fresh herbs

***Method***
Combine ingredients. Mix the dressing and toss, then sprinkle with herbs.

*Cleansing tuna salad*

This can be eaten for lunch on alternate days to the cleansing chicken salad. You can pack this into a glass container and take it with you to work. If any of these foods upset your gut, leave them out or substitute with foods that you can tolerate.

### Ingredients (serves 2)
- 250 gm canned tuna
- 2 tablespoons cooked brown rice
- ½ cup steamed broccolini
- ½ cup baby spinach leaves
- ½ cup chopped cucumber
- ½ cup chopped carrot

### Dressing
- Lemon juice or apple cider vinegar
- Cold-pressed extra virgin olive oil
- Pepper
- Chopped fresh herbs

### Method
Combine ingredients. Mix the dressing and toss, then sprinkle with herbs.

# Dinner recipes

*Cleansing fish*

***Ingredients (serves 2)***
- 300 gm fresh salmon, tuna or white fish
- 1 teaspoon tamarind paste
- Juice of 1 lime
- Sea salt and cracked pepper
- 1 knob diced fresh ginger
- 1 teaspoon coconut oil

***Method***
Rub the fish fillets in a mixture of tamarind paste, lime juice and chilli. Season with salt and pepper. Lightly pan sear the fresh ginger. Add the fish, skin side down, in coconut oil then turn to cook the other side. Serve with steamed vegetables.

*Cleansing meat*

***Ingredients (serves 2)***
- 2 x 250 gm organic grass-fed steaks
- Sea salt and cracked pepper
- 1 teaspoon coconut oil

***Method***
Season the meat with salt and pepper. Lightly pan sear the steaks in coconut oil. Serve with steamed vegetables.

*Steamed vegetables*

### Ingredients
- ½ cup chopped broccoli
- ½ cup sweet potato
- ½ cup chopped zucchini
- ½ cup baby Brussels sprouts
- ¼ cup diced parsley
- ¼ cup diced basil
- 1 tablespoon olive oil
- Juice of 1 lime
- Sea salt and cracked pepper

### Method
Place vegetables in a steamer and cook until soft. Sprinkle with the herbs. Season with olive oil, lime juice, sea salt and cracked pepper.

# Recipes: Microbiome reload diet

## Bone broth

The essential components of a good bone broth are bones, fat, meat, vegetables and water. You can make bone broth with just animal products, but adding vegetables is more beneficial. Use bones from grass-fed animals that are free of antibiotics and hormones. Buy them from your local farmers market or an organic butcher. If you're making beef or lamb broth, brown the meat in a pan before putting it into the pot. Fish and poultry can be added without browning first.

A slow and long cooking time is necessary in order to fully extract the nutrients in and around the bone. Some people like to use feet, ligaments, internal organs and/or the head and boil for 24-48 hours. That's great for unlocking maximum nutrients, but it's very labour intensive. You will still end up with a nutrient-rich bone broth if you follow these recipes.

*Easy chicken bone broth*

### Ingredients

- 1 whole organic free-range chicken
- 1 tablespoon organic apple cider vinegar
- 1 cup chopped onion, carrot and/or celery
- 1 pinch iodised salt

### Method

Place the chicken in a large pot and fill to the top with filtered water. Add the vegetables, apple cider vinegar and salt. Boil for 50 minutes then cool. Remove the chicken and store the broth and vegetables in glass containers for drinking. Pull the meat off the chicken and store separately. As the broth cools, a layer of fat will harden on top. This layer protects the broth. Discard the fat only when you are about to eat the broth. Add some meat to the broth when you serve it.

*Hard-core bone broth*

### Ingredients
- 4 cups of bones, including a joint with cartilage, that have some meat on them
- 2 cups chopped vegetables (e.g. onions, carrots, potato and celery)
- 2 tablespoons organic apple cider vinegar
- Salt and pepper

### Method
Place bones, vegetables and apple cider vinegar into a large stockpot or saucepan. Fill the pot with filtered water. Add salt and pepper to taste. Heat slowly until boiling, then reduce heat to a low simmer. Cook for at least six hours. Remove scum as it rises. Pour off the liquid broth and store in the fridge. Discard bones.

# Breakfast recipes

*Scott's probiotic natural yoghurt*

This recipe for a natural, organic, probiotic-rich, chemical-free yoghurt was given to me by a patient. It works every time.

*Ingredients*
- Enough organic grass-fed milk to fill a yoghurt maker
- Yoghurt starter
  - 125 ml (½ cup) commercial yoghurt starter or homemade natural yoghurt with no additives (e.g. gums, sweeteners, flavours, sugars). It must contain active (live) bacterial cultures. *Lactobacillus delbrueckii* subsp. *bulgaricus*, *Streptococcus thermophilus* and *Lactobacillus acidophilus* are recommended. Multiple sources advise against yoghurt containing *Bifidobacterium bifidum*.

or

  - Live culture (follow the directions about quantity and note the recommended strains discussed above). These can be bought online from greenlivingaustralia.com.au (mild dairy yoghurt starter) or shop.gapsaustralia.com.au (GI ProStart).

*Equipment*
- Saucepan
- Measuring jug
- Stainless steel spoons
- Thermometer (suitable for use with food)
- Yoghurt maker

*Method*
- Rinse all equipment with boiling water.
- Heat milk in saucepan (stir constantly to prevent scorching) to above 72°C for at least 15 seconds. Avoid boiling the milk.
- Remove pan from heat and cool to 35-40° C.
- Pour a little of the milk into the yoghurt maker. Add yoghurt starter or live culture. Stir thoroughly until dissolved.
- Add remainder of the cooled milk and stir thoroughly.
- Switch yoghurt maker on and select temperature (40°C seems to work well).
- Do not move the yoghurt maker, remove the lid or the stir contents during the incubation period as this might cause the mixture to curdle.

- When the incubation period is complete (ideally up to 24 hours for low lactose yoghurt), refrigerate for a minimum of 8 hours to achieve a firmly set yoghurt.
- Stir before serving as it tends to separate over time.
- Yoghurt will keep refrigerated for up to two weeks.

*Stewed apple and cinnamon*

Stewed apple is easy to make. Adding cinnamon slows the absorption of the sugars from the stewed apple, which makes it a lower GI food. Using sour apples is also fine, but you may want to add a few raisins or dates to sweeten. Stewing the apple also releases pectin, especially if you leave some of the skin on. If the apples are not organic, make sure you clean the skin with hot water and a towel before cooking.

*Ingredients (4 serves)*
- 4 apples, cored, partially peeled and chopped
- 4 tablespoons filtered water
- 2 teaspoons cinnamon

*Method*
Put apples and water into a pan. Heat until lightly boiling, then add cinnamon. Cook for 8-10 minutes, until apples are soft. Take off the heat and refrigerate.

*Omelette with spinach and lemon kale*

**Ingredients**
- 2 organic eggs
- 1 tablespoon filtered water
- 1 teaspoon organic grass-fed butter
- 1 cup baby spinach leaves
- 1 cup chopped kale
- Juice of 1/2 lemon
- Olive oil
- Salt and pepper

**Method:**
Heat olive oil and sauté the spinach and kale until soft. Set aside and keep warm. Crack the eggs into a bowl with water. Add salt and pepper to taste. Whisk until fluffy. Melt butter in a fry pan then pour in the egg mixture. Cook for two minutes then fold in half. Drizzle the sautéed greens with lemon juice and season with salt and pepper. Serve the omelette with the greens on the side.

*Grilled mushroom salad*

**Ingredients**
- ½ cup mixed mushrooms, chopped
- 1 tablespoon feta cheese
- 1 cup rocket leaves
- 1 roma tomato, halved
- Olive oil

**Method**
Grill the mushrooms and tomato. Crumble the feta on top of the mushrooms. Serve on a bed of rocket and top with tomato.

*Poached eggs on quinoa and vegetables*

***Ingredients***
- 2 organic eggs, poached
- ½ cup cooked organic quinoa
- ½ cup cooked cauliflower, chopped
- ½ cooked onion
- ½ cup cooked asparagus, chopped
- Olive oil
- Lemon juice

***Method***
Place the poached eggs on a bed of quinoa, asparagus, cauliflower and onion. Dress with olive oil and lemon juice and season with and salt and pepper.

*Ancestral muesli*

You can purchase Paleo muesli from your local health food store or make it yourself at home.

***Method***
A simple ancestral muesli can be made by mixing together equal parts of chopped activated almonds, hazelnuts, walnuts, chia seeds, macadamias, pepitas, coconut shavings and cacao nibs.

*Fruit salad with coconut*

**Ingredients**
- ¼ rockmelon, sliced
- 1 kiwi fruit, sliced
- 1 apple, sliced
- 1 tablespoon blackberries
- 1 tablespoon shredded coconut
- Juice of ½ lemon
- 1 tablespoon probiotic yoghurt
- 1 tablespoon kefir
- 1 tablespoon flaxseed meal

**Method**

In a bowl, mix fruit, coconut and lemon juice. Top with 1 tablespoon yoghurt, 1 tablespoon kefir and 1 tablespoon flaxseed meal.

*Ancestral porridge*

**Ingredients**
- 1 tablespoon cooked quinoa
- 1 tablespoon cooked buckwheat
- 1 tablespoon cooked rolled oats
- 1 tablespoon almond milk
- 1 teaspoon chopped almonds
- 2 strawberries or raspberries, chopped
- 1 date, chopped
- 1 tablespoon probiotic yoghurt

**Method**

Mix quinoa, buckwheat and rolled oats. Add almond milk and heat in a saucepan until warm. Sprinkle with chopped almonds, dates, strawberries or raspberries and yoghurt.

## Green smoothie bowl

### Ingredients
- ½ cup baby spinach leaves
- 1 kiwi fruit, peeled
- ½ cup frozen mango
- 1 scoop vanilla protein powder
- 1 tablespoon coconut water
- 1 tablespoon coconut shavings
- juice of ½ lime
- 1 teaspoon pepitas
- 1 tablespoon blueberries

### Method
Blend ingredients in a blender or NutriBullet until smooth. Top with pepitas and blueberries.

## Green cacao shake

### Ingredients
- ¼ cup kale
- ¼ cup baby spinach leaves
- 1 scoop chocolate protein powder
- 1 teaspoon organic cacao powder
- 1 tablespoon frozen cherries
- 1 teaspoon chia seeds
- ½ frozen banana
- 1 cup almond milk
- 1 teaspoon kefir yoghurt
- 2 cubes ice

### Method
Blend ingredients in a blender or NutriBullet until smooth.

*Almond banana smoothie*

**Ingredients**
- ½ cup almond milk
- 1 teaspoon almond meal
- 1 scoop vanilla protein powder
- 1 frozen banana
- 1 teaspoon chia seeds
- 1 tablespoon frozen mango
- Juice of ½ lemon
- 4 strawberries, quartered
- ½ cup almonds, chopped

**Method**

Blend ingredients in a blender or NutriBullet until smooth. Top with strawberries and almonds.

# Lunch recipes

*Tuna and green salad*

### Ingredients
- ½ cup baby spinach leaves
- ½ cup baby beetroot leaves
- ½ cup broccoli, steamed
- ½ cup zucchini, steamed
- 125g tuna (fresh grilled or tinned in brine)
- 1 teaspoon walnuts, chopped
- 1 teaspoon goji berries
- 1 teaspoon lemon juice
- 1 teaspoon extra virgin olive oil

### Method
In a bowl, mix together spinach and beetroot leaves, broccoli and zucchini. Serve the tuna on top of the salad and sprinkle with walnuts and goji berries. Dress with a squeeze of lemon juice and 1 tsp extra virgin olive oil.

*Chicken soup with avocado salad*

### Ingredients
- 1 cup chicken bone broth
- ½ cup shredded chicken and vegetables from broth recipe
- ½ cup cos lettuce
- ½ cup radicchio lettuce
- 1 baby beetroot, cooked
- ½ avocado
- 1 teaspoon red wine vinegar
- 1 teaspoon olive oil

### Method
Heat broth and add chicken and vegetables. Toss lettuce, beetroot and avocado with red wine vinegar and olive oil.

*Vegetable stack*

**Ingredients**
- ½ eggplant, sliced and grilled
- 1 capsicum, sliced, deseeded and grilled
- 1 slice of sweet potato, steamed
- ½ cup baby spinach, blanched
- 1 slice of zucchini, grilled
- 1 bocconcini, sliced
- ½ cup Napoli sauce
- 1 pinch sauerkraut
- 1 tablespoon chopped fresh basil

**Method**
Stack vegetables and bocconcini in layers. Drizzle with Napoli sauce and top with sauerkraut and basil.

*Beef soup with baked sweet potato*

**Ingredients**
- 1 cup beef bone broth
- ½ cup shredded beef and vegetables from broth recipe
- ½ sweet potato, baked
- 1 tablespoon probiotic yoghurt
- 1 tablespoon slivered activated almonds

**Method**
Heat the beef broth and add beef and vegetables. Serve with baked sweet potato topped with yoghurt and almonds.

*Salmon and rocket salad*

**Ingredients**
- 150g salmon (fresh or tinned)
- 1 cup rocket
- ½ pear, sliced
- 1 tablespoon pecans, chopped
- Juice of 1 lemon
- ½ cup cooked buckwheat
- ½ avocado, chopped
- 1 teaspoon kimchi

**Method**
Grill the salmon and serve on the rocket, pear and pecans. Drizzle with lemon juice. Mix the buckwheat, avocado and kimchi and serve on the side.

*Chicken soup with cucumber salad*

**Ingredients**
- 1 cup chicken bone broth
- ½ cup shredded cooked chicken and vegetables from broth recipe
- 1 Lebanese cucumber, sliced
- ¼ Spanish onion, sliced
- 1 teaspoon capers
- pinch of paprika
- red wine vinegar

**Method**
Heat the chicken broth and add shredded chicken and vegetables. Mix cucumber, onion, capers, paprika and vinegar and serve on the side.

*Grilled chicken with rice and vegetables*

**Ingredients**
- 200 gm chicken breast
- Pinch paprika
- Salt and pepper
- ½ cup brown rice, cooked
- 2 spring onions, chopped
- ½ cup broccolini, steamed and chopped
- ½ cup asparagus, steamed
- 1 teaspoon Kalamata olives, chopped
- 1 teaspoon kimchi

**Method**

Season the chicken with salt, pepper and paprika, then grill. Serve on a bed of rice mixed with broccolini, asparagus, spring onion, olives, and kimchi.

*Minestrone with fennel and orange salad*

**Ingredients**
- 1 cup minestrone soup
- ½ cup baby fennel bulb, thinly sliced
- ½ cup mixed red oak lettuce and rocket
- 1 orange, peeled and segmented
- 2 radishes, chopped
- 1 teaspoon olive oil
- 1 teaspoon red wine vinegar
- 1 teaspoon orange juice

**Method**

Heat the minestrone. Mix the lettuce, rocket, fennel, radish and orange segments. Dress with olive oil, red wine vinegar and orange juice.

*Beef soup with mixed vegetables*

**Ingredients**
- 1 cup beef bone broth
- ½ cup shredded beef from broth recipe
- 1 cup cauliflower florets
- 1 teaspoon coconut oil
- 3 asparagus spears, steamed
- ⅓ cup broccolini, steamed
- 1 teaspoon almonds, chopped
- ½ peach, sliced
- 1 teaspoon sauerkraut

**Method**
Heat the beef broth with shredded beef. Place cauliflower in a food processor and process for 15 seconds or until it resembles rice. Cook in a pan with coconut oil for five minutes until semi-soft. Mix with asparagus, broccolini, almonds and peaches and top with sauerkraut.

*Baked sweet potato salad*

**Ingredients**
- ½ sweet potato
- 1 tablespoon probiotic yoghurt
- 1 teaspoon walnuts, chopped
- ½ cup baby spinach leaves
- ½ cup cos lettuce
- ½ capsicum, deseeded and sliced
- 1 radish, sliced
- 1 tablespoon green olives

**Method**
Peel sweet potato, slice lengthways and bake in the oven at 160°C until soft. Mix the spinach, cos lettuce, capsicum, radish and green olives. Top the baked sweet potato with yoghurt and walnuts and serve.

# Dinner recipes

*Spinach and radicchio salad*

### Ingredients
- ½ cup baby spinach leaves
- ½ cup radicchio lettuce, chopped
- ¼ cup green capsicum, chopped
- ¼ cup parsley, chopped
- 1 teaspoon extra virgin olive oil
- 1 teaspoon organic apple cider vinegar

### Method
Mix the spinach, radicchio, capsicum and parsley. Dress with olive oil and vinegar.

*Pesto chicken and vegetables*

### Ingredients
- 1 cup firmly packed fresh basil leaves
- ¼ cup pine nuts
- ½ cup parmesan cheese, grated
- 4 tablespoons extra virgin olive oil
- 200g organic free-range chicken fillet
- ½ cup broccolini
- ½ cup cauliflower, chopped
- ½ cup pumpkin, chopped
- 1 tablespoon walnuts, chopped
- 1 teaspoon sauerkraut

### Method
Make the pesto by placing the basil, pine nuts, cheese and olive oil into a food processor and processing until smooth. It can be stored in the fridge until you need it. Season the chicken fillet with salt and pepper then grill until cooked. Steam the vegetables and add walnuts and sauerkraut. Top the chicken and vegetables with 1 tablespoon of the pesto.

*Beetroot, rocket and cabbage salad*

**Ingredients**
- ½ cup baby beetroot leaves
- ½ cup rocket, chopped
- ¼ cup cabbage, chopped
- ¼ cup cucumber, chopped
- 1 teaspoon kimchi
- 1 teaspoon extra virgin olive oil
- 1 teaspoon organic apple cider vinegar

**Method**
Mix the beetroot leaves, rocket, cabbage, kimchi and cucumber. Dress olive oil and vinegar.

*Steak and winter vegetables*

**Ingredients**
- 250 gm grass-fed steak
- ½ cup sweet potato
- ½ cup carrot
- ½ cup turnip
- ½ cup pumpkin

**Method**
Chop vegetables and dry roast them in the oven at 180°C until soft. Season steak with salt and pepper and grill until medium-rare.

*Spinach and kale salad*

**Ingredients**
- ½ cup baby spinach leaves
- ½ cup kale, chopped
- 1 teaspoon sauerkraut
- 1 teaspoon sesame seeds
- 1 teaspoon extra virgin olive oil
- 1 teaspoon organic apple cider vinegar

**Method**
Mix spinach leaves, kale, sauerkraut and sesame seeds. Dress with olive oil and vinegar.

*Chilli ginger prawns*

**Ingredients**
- 200 gm king prawns
- 2 teaspoons coconut oil
- 1 clove garlic, crushed
- 1 teaspoon fresh ginger, chopped
- 1 red chilli, chopped
- 1 carrot, julienned
- 1 baby beetroot, chopped
- ½ cup cooked brown rice

**Method**
Sauté the prawns in coconut oil with garlic, ginger and chilli. Serve with carrot, beetroot and rice.

*Spinach, celery and cabbage salad*

**Ingredients**
- ½ cup baby spinach leaves
- ¼ stick celery, chopped
- ¼ cup purple cabbage, chopped
- Juice of ½ lime

**Method**
Mix spinach, celery and cabbage. Drizzle with lime juice.

*Fish and cauliflower rice*

**Ingredients**
- 150 gm white fish fillet
- 1 clove garlic
- 1 stick lemongrass, chopped
- 1 knob of fresh ginger
- 1 teaspoon tamari
- 1 cup cauliflower florets
- 1 teaspoon coconut oil
- 1 tablespoon fresh coriander
- 1 teaspoon walnuts, chopped

**Method**
Place the fish in foil and top with garlic, lemongrass, ginger and tamari. Bake in the oven at 160°C for 10 minutes. Place cauliflower in a food processor and process for 15 seconds or until it resembles rice. Cook in a pan with coconut oil for five minutes until semi-soft. Serve the fish on top of the cauliflower rice and sprinkle with walnuts and coriander.

*Spinach, kale and red oak salad*

**Ingredients**
- ½ cup red oak lettuce
- ½ cup baby spinach leaves
- ¼ cup chopped kale
- 1 teaspoon extra virgin olive oil
- 1 teaspoon red wine vinegar.

**Method**
Mix leaves and dress with olive oil and vinegar.

*Roast lamb and winter vegetables*

**Ingredients**
- 200 gm grass-fed lamb fillet
- ½ cup baby Brussels sprouts
- ½ cup sweet potato, chopped
- ½ cup turnip, chopped
- 1 leek, chopped
- 1 sprig of rosemary

**Method**
Sear the lamb on all sides in a pan then place in an oven dish with rosemary and vegetables. Bake at 180°C until cooked.

*Cos, endive and kale salad*

**Ingredients**
- ½ cup cos lettuce
- ¼ cup endive
- ¼ cup kale, chopped
- 1 teaspoon walnuts, chopped
- 1 teaspoon extra virgin olive oil
- 1 teaspoon lemon juice

**Method**
Mix the leaves and dress with olive oil and lemon juice.

*Zucchini noodles with meatballs and Napoli sauce*

**Ingredients**
- 2 large zucchini
- 1 teaspoon coconut oil
- 1 cup homemade meatballs (use grass-fed mince), cooked
- 1 cup homemade Napoli sauce
- 2 Roma tomatoes
- 2 bocconcini balls
- 1 teaspoon fresh basil, chopped

**Method**
Shred the zucchini with a mandolin to make noodles. Lightly cook the noodles in a pan of coconut oil for 3 minutes or until soft. Heat the meatballs in the Napoli sauce. Mix the noodles with the meatballs and sauce. Serve with bocconcini, tomatoes and basil.

*Spinach, rocket and pear salad*

**Ingredients**
- ½ cup baby spinach
- ½ cup rocket
- ½ pear, sliced
- 1 teaspoon almonds
- 1 teaspoon extra virgin olive oil
- 1 teaspoon balsamic vinegar

**Method**
Combine spinach, rocket and pear. Top with almonds and drizzle with olive oil and vinegar.

*Tamarind and lime salmon with vegetables*

**Ingredients**
- Salmon fillet 200g
- 1 clove crushed garlic
- Juice of ½ a lime
- 1 teaspoon tamarind paste
- ½ cup broccoli, steamed
- ½ cup snow peas, steamed
- ½ cup pumpkin, chopped and steamed
- Chilli salt

**Method**
Combine the garlic, lime juice and tamarind paste. Coat one side of the salmon fillet with the mixture and grill, turning once. Served with broccolini, snow peas and pumpkin, seasoned with chilli salt.

*Spinach and beetroot salad*

***Ingredients***
- ½ cup baby spinach leaves
- ½ baby beetroot leaves
- 1 teaspoon sauerkraut
- 1 teaspoon extra virgin olive oil
- 1 teaspoon balsamic vinegar

***Method***
Mix leaves and sauerkraut. Dress with olive oil and vinegar.

*Chicken stir fry*

***Ingredients***
- 200 gm organic free-range chicken breast, chopped
- 1 tablespoon tamari
- 1 garlic clove, crushed
- ½ onion, chopped
- 1 knob ginger, chopped
- 1 chilli, chopped
- 2 teaspoons coconut oil
- ⅓cup broccoli, chopped
- ⅓ cup carrot, chopped
- ⅓ cup asparagus, chopped
- ⅓ cup capsicum, chopped
- ⅓ cup bean shoots
- 1 tablespoon oyster sauce
- 1 teaspoon fish sauce
- 1 cup cauliflower florets
- ½ cup bok choy, steamed

***Method***
Season the chicken with tamari. Cook lightly in a wok and put aside. Place cauliflower in a food processor and process for 15 seconds or until it resembles rice. Cook in a pan with coconut oil for five minutes until semi-soft. Put aside. Stir fry the garlic, onion, ginger and chilli in 1 teaspoon of the coconut oil for 2 minutes. Add chicken, broccoli, carrot, asparagus, capsicum and bean shoots and fry until chicken is cooked. When almost ready, drizzle in a mixture of tamari, oyster sauce and fish sauce. Serve with cauliflower rice and steamed bok choy.

*Spinach and butter lettuce salad*

**Ingredients**
- ½ cup baby spinach
- ½ cup butter lettuce
- ¼ cup parsley
- 1 teaspoon extra virgin olive oil
- 1 teaspoon lemon juice.

**Method**
Combine spinach, lettuce and parsley and dress with oil and lemon juice.

*Tuna with wasabi mash*

**Ingredients**
- 250 gm tuna fillet
- ½ cup pumpkin
- ½ cup potato
- 1 knob organic butter
- 1 teaspoon wasabi
- ½ onion
- 1 teaspoon coconut oil
- ½ cup broccolini, steamed
- ½ cup baby Brussels sprouts, steamed

**Method**
Peel and chop pumpkin and potato. Boil until soft, then mash with butter and wasabi. Shallow-fry onion in coconut oil. Season the tuna and grill until medium-rare. Serve tuna on a bed of mash with steamed broccolini and Brussels sprouts and top with onion.

*Kale, parsley and parmesan salad*

**Ingredients**
- ½ cup kale, chopped
- ½ cup parsley, chopped
- ½ cup parmesan cheese, grated
- 1 tablespoon almonds, toasted and diced
- 1 teaspoon extra virgin olive oil
- 1 teaspoon lemon juice

**Method**
Toss kale, parsley, parmesan and almonds. Drizzle with olive oil and lemon juice.

*Eggplant parmigiana*

**Ingredients**
- 1 eggplant, cut into 1 cm slices
- 1 tablespoon extra virgin olive oil
- ½ onion, diced
- 1 clove garlic, chopped
- 1 tablespoon tomato paste
- 2 Roma tomatoes
- ½ cup Napoli sauce
- 1 tablespoon fresh basil
- 1 tablespoon parmesan cheese, grated

**Method**
Salt the eggplant slices, then rinse in cold water and pat dry with a paper towel. Cook eggplant in a pan with olive oil until soft. Put aside. Sauté onion and garlic until transparent. Add tomato paste, tomato, basil and ½ cup water and simmer until smooth. Layer eggplant with parmesan cheese and Napoli sauce. Bake in oven for 20 minutes at 160 °C. Serve with parmesan.

# Shopping list

A shopping list is helpful because it encourages you to buy healthy food. It makes it easy to fill your fridge and kitchen cupboards with healthy alternatives to junk food. When you're hungry, you can open the pantry or fridge to find shelves stacked with nuts, seeds, fruit and vegetables you will want to eat. Where possible, buy organic. Always look for fresh, seasonal fruit and vegetables. Read this list and highlight the items you are going to bring back into your life.

*Vegetables*
Choose a range of the following: capsicum, mushrooms, broccolini, broccoli, rocket, red oak lettuce, cos lettuce, endive, spring onion, baby beetroot, carrot, avocado, snow peas, bean shoots, onions, garlic, pumpkin, zucchini, bok choy, baby spinach leaves, baby beetroot leaves, leeks, sweet potato, turnips, red cabbage, asparagus, parsley, coriander.

*Fruit*
Choose a wide range. Fresh is best but the most convenient will often be frozen. Phytonutrient-packed fruits include blueberries, raspberries, blackberries, kiwi fruit and strawberries. Dried fruit should be kept to a minimum – no more than ¼ of a cup a day. Choose goji berries, figs, prunes, dates and sultanas. Small amounts only of mango and watermelon (because of the very high fructose content). Avoid mixed fruit balls and processed muesli or fruit bars.

*Seeds and nuts*
Activated almonds, walnuts, flax seed meal, chia seeds and LSA mix.

*Meat and fish*
When you can, choose organic free-range chicken or turkey. Lamb fillets are lean with very little fat. Fish such as tuna, salmon, snapper, barramundi, cod, perch or whiting. Good-quality canned fish such as tuna, sardines, salmon or herring can be used on occasions. Avoid crumbed fish. Steer clear of swordfish and flake – these large fish have the highest mercury content. No processed meats (e.g. sausages, bacon, salami, devon) or processed meat substitutes such as soy sausages. No smoked fish or fish substitutes.

*Eggs*
Free-range eggs are best.

*Grains*

Purchase brown rice, wild rice, buckwheat, whole organic oats, quinoa and spelt. Avoid wheat, rye and barley products such as pasta, noodles, cakes, doughnuts, buns and pastries. No bread or biscuits, even gluten-free ones.

*Dairy*

Use only natural probiotic yoghurt, parmesan and bocconcini cheese and grass-fed butter.

*Legumes*

Chick peas, lentils, green beans, black beans and cannelloni beans can be eaten on occasions.

*Breakfast cereals*

Rice flakes, puffed quinoa, organic (unsweetened) paleo muesli. Mix LSA (linseed, sunflower and almonds), organic shaved coconut and almond meal into the cereals. Lecithin granules can also be put onto gluten-free cereals. Avoid all processed wheat or corn-based cereals as they are full of sugar.

*Snacks*

Sunflower seeds, pumpkin seeds. Eat rice cakes, rice crackers and dried fruit in moderation.

*Herbal tea*

Green tea (no milk or sugar), peppermint, lemon and ginger, chamomile.

*Oils*

Extra virgin olive oil and coconut oil are great, but avoid all margarines and seed oils.

*Sauces*

Good quality tamari is a healthy substitute for soy sauce. Avoid all other sauces, mustards, pickles and commercial dressings.

*Dressings*

Use extra virgin olive oil with a squeeze of lemon, balsamic vinegar, red wine vinegar or organic apple cider vinegar.

*Other flavours*

Ground nutmeg, cinnamon, basil, coriander, thyme, marjoram, sea salt, kaffir lime leaves.

CPSIA information can be obtained
at www.ICGtesting.com
Printed in the USA
BVHW062009170519
548593BV00006B/93/P

9 781921 919923